FICTION AND FANTASY
IN MEDICAL RESEARCH

The Large-Scale Randomised Trial

James Penston

The
London
Press

Copyright © 2003 by James Penston
Published in the United Kingdom by The London Press Ltd.
Cover by Mary Helen Fein of Parallax Design Group
(www.parallaxdesigngroup.com)

British Library Cataloguing in Publication Data

Penston, James
Fiction and fantasy in medical research : the large scale randomised trial
1.Clinical trials 2.Clinical trials – Evaluation
I .Title
615.5'0724

ISBN 0954463617

To Rebecca, Victoria and Fiona

Contents

I

THE GOLD STANDARD OF MEDICAL RESEARCH? - SCRATCHING THE SURFACE

The elderly woman settles into her bed on the admission ward. Throughout her life, medicine has been good to her. Sixty years ago, a prompt caesarean section saved the life of her first-born; in her fifties, thyroxine restored her to health; after her retirement, a total hip replacement transformed her crippled existence into an independent, pain-free life of an active senior citizen; and, a decade later, cataract surgery gave her back her sight. Without doubt, she is a testament to the enormous advances in medicine which occurred throughout the twentieth century. Yet, on the other hand, she also bears witness to the more dubious side of medical research. In response to the doctor's enquiry about her current medication, she struggles to lift a plastic carrier bag from the top of the locker and tips the contents onto the bed. There are eleven different pills and capsules in a mixture of bottles and blister packs, two inhalers, a large bottle of pink liquid, a spray dispenser and a tube of cream. The picture is familiar to all who are involved in the care of patients throughout the country. So, too, is the elderly woman's aside that the concoction of pills and potions does not seem to be of much benefit. And, in the face of her recurrent admissions over the past few years, the doctor's assurance that her medication is of proven value has a hollow ring about it. Just how secure is the knowledge that these drugs will improve her health?

The Gold Standard of Medical Research?

The conventional reply to such questions is that the efficacy of drugs has been established by randomised controlled trials. This methodology is universally recognised as the gold standard in medical research – if a drug has been shown to be of benefit in a randomised study, then its efficacy is all but beyond dispute. For more than fifty years, the randomised trial has captured the imagination of medical scientists and clinicians alike, and the results from this type of study have become generally accepted as the most reliable form of medical knowledge: *"Randomised clinical trials are rightfully regarded as the best tools for gathering evidence on the effectiveness of health care interventions."* [1] Guidelines issued by the Royal Colleges, for example, regularly include a statement giving the greatest credence to evidence provided by randomised trials while medical journals treat this methodology with the utmost reverence - in 1998 the *British Medical Journal* dedicated an entire issue in celebration of the fiftieth birthday of the randomised controlled trial.

Such is the devotion to the randomised trial that it borders on heresy even to question its status as the provider of the purest form of medical knowledge. When the *New England Journal of Medicine* published two papers which suggested that observational studies produced results equivalent to those of randomised controlled trials,[2,3] the response was swift and uncompromising: *"If high quality randomised controlled trials exist for a clinical question then they trump any number of observational studies."* [4] This exaggerated confidence in the methodology of research is not, however, restricted to medicine. In *The Structure of Scientific Revolutions,*[5] Thomas Kuhn drew attention to the way in which the basic features of any scientific endeavour – the paradigm – are not open to question by those involved in the research. This observation applies no less to randomised trials. The methodology is so deeply ingrained that questions about its validity never surface. Yet there are reasons to believe that it is, nonetheless, flawed.

During the past 20 years, there has been a trend in favour of larger and larger randomised trials. This reflects both the limited knowledge of diseases and the low efficacy of many newly developed drugs. For example, if there is insufficient information to identify a subgroup of patients with hypertension who would develop cerebro-vascular disease, then all patients with hypertension have to be included in clinical trials investigating anti-hypertensive drugs to prevent strokes. This, combined with the expectation that the drugs are effective in preventing strokes in only a minority of patients within the subgroup, necessitates the recruitment of very large numbers of patients in order to show a statistical difference in outcome between the active drug and the control group. These conditions account for the current fashion for large randomised controlled trials, or mega-trials, involving many thousands of patients. It is, however, these large randomised trials that raise the most serious questions about current medical research.

Given the widespread acceptance of large-scale randomised trials, it is salutary to note the frequent disputes that arise regarding their conclusions. For example, arguments relating to the value of mammography in breast cancer,[6] of thrombolytic therapy in strokes[7,8] and of long-term aspirin therapy in ischaemic heart disease[9,10] have all involved the interpretation of randomised trials. If the methodology really is secure, how are such disputes to be explained?

The thesis presented in this text is that large-scale randomised trials are deeply flawed. Errors in the design, execution and analysis of randomised trials are commonplace; literature reviews have repeatedly shown that the standard of published trials leaves much scope for improvement. The small treatment differences characteristic of mega-trials have little relevance to individual patients while the vast majority of those who receive treatment based on the results of these studies obtain no benefit whatsoever. Furthermore, claims that the results of mega-trials yield major improvements in health when applied to the wider population of patients are highly contentious. At a more fundamental level, the methodology of these studies is without any sound foundation. Whilst it is generally assumed that mega-trials are grounded in the scientific method, the differences between the two are so great as to militate against the assertion that the validity of mega-trials rests on their links with science. And, if mega-trials are not grounded in the scientific method, then the validity of the methodology must be established independently – a task which, given the nature of the data, has no readily forthcoming solution.

These criticisms of large-scale clinical trials have significant consequences for patients, the medical profession and those charged with the delivery of health-care. Treating patients on the basis of the results of mega-trials leads to a waste of scarce health-care resources and the unnecessary exposure of large numbers of patients to adverse drug reactions. The ethical implications, especially with respect to the information provided to patients, cannot be ignored. The ease with which the data from mega-trials are manipulated is of great concern, as, too, is the absence of any satisfactory controls against research fraud; this is particularly important given that drugs investigated by these studies are designed for use in the common, chronic diseases afflicting western societies and, thus, have the potential for creating enormous profits for pharmaceutical companies. In this context, an awareness of the influence of those with a vested interest in the outcome of mega-trials is crucial to any objective assessment of the results.

Anyone who has not been indoctrinated with the orthodox approach to medical research could be forgiven for reacting to the results of a large-scale randomised trial with a mixture of bemusement and incredulity. They could be forgiven, too, for wondering why so much fuss was being made about something with so little substance. And they could be forgiven for feeling highly suspicious about the almost mystical tricks of the statisticians. Anyone with an ounce of healthy scepticism would surely agree that the time has come to subject the large-scale randomised trial to rigorous scrutiny.

References

1. Bossuyt PMM. Better standards for better reporting of RCTs. *Br Med J* 2001;322;1317-8.

2. Benson K & Hartz AJ. A comparison of observational and randomised, controlled trials. *N Eng J Med* 2000;342;1878-86.

3. Concato J, Shah N, Horwitz RI. Randomised, controlled trials, observational studies, and the hierarchy of research designs. *N Eng J Med* 2000;342;1887-92.

4. Barton S. Which clinical studies provide the best evidence? *Br Med J* 2000;321;255-6.

5. Kuhn T. *The Structure of Scientific Revolutions.* University of Chicago Press; Chicago, 1962.

6. Gelmon KA, & Olivotto I. The mammography screening debate: time to move on. *Lancet* 2002;359;904-5.

7. Lenzer J. Alteplase for stroke: money and optimistic claims buttress the "brain attack" campaign. *Br Med J* 2002;324;723-9.

8. Saver JL, Kidwell CS, Starkman S. Commentary: Thrombolysis in stroke: it works! *Br Med J* 2002;324;727-9.

9. Antithrombotic Trialists' Collaboration. Collaborative meta-analysis of randomised trials of antiplatelet therapy for prevention of death, myocardial infarction, and stroke in high risk patients. *Br Med J* 2002;324;71-86.

10. Cleland JGF. For debate: Preventing atherosclerotic events with aspirin. *Br Med J* 2002;324;103-5.

II

BACON, HUME AND THE SCIENTIFIC METHOD
- LESSONS FROM HISTORY

The randomised controlled trial is a tool for investigating the relationship between one event – for example, the administration of a drug – and another, such as the outcome of a disease. In this respect, it is similar to an experiment in science. Each of the methods aims to provide knowledge of phenomena in the natural world. In particular, their purpose is to produce generalisations which have practical applications. If a generalisation is reliable, then it allows us to act intentionally in such a way as to promote or prevent a specific outcome.

As will be argued repeatedly throughout the text, randomised controlled trials differ from the scientific method in many respects and the flaws inherent in clinical research have their origins in these differences. For any appreciation of the problems arising from randomised trials, it is important that the differences between this methodology and that of science are brought clearly into view.

For centuries, the scientific method has yielded major advances in our knowledge of the world around us. But why are its predictions so accurate and its generalisations so reliable while alternative methods of forecasting – for instance, astrology, crystal ball gazing and tarot card reading – fail to deliver on their promises? The answer, of course, is that science is based on experience which is interpreted in accordance with the principles of induction and causation.

Induction

The world, as we perceive it, displays a certain regularity. Similar objects and similar events recur throughout history. Every morning the sun rises and every evening it sets. Each spring, the flowers blossom and, when autumn arrives, the leaves turn brown and fall to the ground. Rocks dislodged from side of a mountain always role downhill and smoke always rises. It is the observation of such regularities that is the foundation of induction.

Induction is a form of inference, that is, a method of reasoning by which a new proposition is reached on the basis of other propositions. Traditionally, methods of inference have been divided into two types: deduction and induction. In a deductive argument, the conclusion follows logically from the premises alone; if the deductive argument is valid, then, given the truth of the premises, the conclusion is necessarily true.

Deduction	
Premise 1	**All mammals have lungs**
Premise 2	**All sabre-toothed tigers are mammals**
Conclusion	**All sabre-toothed tigers have lungs**

In contrast, an inductive argument does not guarantee the truth of the conclusion; there is no logical necessity involved. Instead, the premises of an inductive argument offer support - of a variable degree - in favour of the conclusion.

7

Induction	
Premise 1	**Sabre-toothed tigers eat cavemen in England**
Premise 2	**Sabre-toothed tigers eat cavemen in Scotland**
Premise 3	**Sabre-toothed tigers eat cavemen in Ireland**
Premise 4	**Sabre-toothed tigers eat cavemen in Wales**
Conclusion	**All sabre-toothed tigers eat cavemen**

Unlike deduction, where the conclusion merely reformulates what is already contained in the premises, induction expands knowledge. The conclusion of an inductive argument contains more information than is present in the premises alone. In the example, the premises provide information about particular instances of sabre-toothed tigers; the conclusion, on the other hand, asserts that all sabre-toothed tigers - not merely those already mentioned – eat cavemen. Hence, this generalisation allows statements to be made about sabre-toothed tigers that have not yet been observed. In other words, the evidence from past instances permits inferences about future instances of the same phenomenon.

For our actions to be purposeful, we need to be able to predict their outcomes. Of course, in our daily lives, we do not ponder the uniformity of nature or dwell on inferences based on induction before we act. It is rather that induction underlies much of our behaviour. When we leave the house in the morning, we give no thought to the solidity of the pavement; it never enters our heads to consider that we might sink into the depths of the earth. But, nevertheless, we know that the pavement will bear our weight and if we were asked to justify this we would do so by mentioning our past experience in similar circumstances, the experience of other people, our knowledge of the qualities of concrete, and many other related facts. This does not mean that we never overtly use inductive thinking in everyday life. For example, if every packet of cornflakes bought each week from a particular shop for the past month has been mouldy, we would shop elsewhere and justify the decision by saying that experience suggested that future cornflakes from the original shop would also be mouldy.

But, despite the ease with which we accept the validity of inductive inference, it nevertheless remains justifiable to question the foundation of such reasoning. Does induction yield knowledge? Are the generalisations reached on the basis of observations instances completely reliable? These questions were first addressed in the Age of the Enlightenment. It is characteristic of philosophy that it asks deep questions, questions that trouble us, questions that strike at the very foundations of our beliefs. And few philosophers have asked more disturbing questions than David Hume (1711-1776). In his great philosophical works - *A Treatise of Human Nature*[1] and *An Enquiry concerning Human Understanding*[2] - he dissected out the bare bones of induction and causation, exposing the insubstantial basis of scientific thinking and leaving scholars troubled and perplexed for more than two centuries. Induction, as discussed above, involves the inference from premises relating to particular observation instances to a conclusion which is a generalisation and applies to all instances of the phenomenon, past, present and future. But, Hume did not accept this inference at face value and he sought to enquire into the justification for induction.

Firstly, he argued that induction is not logically necessary. *"We can at least conceive a change in the course of nature; which sufficiently proves, that such a change is not absolutely impossible. To form a clear idea of anything, is an undeniable argument for its possibility, and is alone a refutation of any pretended demonstration against it."* [3] Given any generalisation, we can imagine a situation which contradicts it; as it is impossible to picture an illogical situation, the imagined situation must be logically possible; hence, the generalisation cannot be logically necessary. Put simply, the inference from particular observation statements to a generalisation is not based on logic. This is clearly shown in the case of the generalisation "all swans are white": no matter how many observations supported this generalisation, it remained logically possible - long before the discovery of black swans in Western Australia - that a swan existed that was yellow or pink or any other colour.

Secondly, Hume argued that induction cannot be justified by reference to previous experience. *"But you must confess that the inference is not intuitive; neither is it demonstrative: Of what nature is it, then? To say it is experimental, is begging the question. For all inferences from experience suppose, as their foundation, that the future will resemble the past... It is impossible, therefore, that any arguments from experience can prove this resemblance of the past to the future; since all arguments are founded on the supposition of that resemblance."* [4] The circularity involved in any argument justifying induction on the grounds of its successful application in the past is, perhaps, most readily appreciated in schematic form:

The Circular Argument for Induction	
Instance 1	Observations report water boils at 100^0C Hence, all water boils at 100^0C
Premise 1	**Induction shown to work successfully**
Instance 2	Observations report acid turns blue litmus red Hence, all acid turns blue litmus red
Premise 2	**Induction shown to work successfully**
Instance 3	Observations report that dogs have kidneys Hence, all dogs have kidneys
Premise 3	**Induction shown to work successfully**
Conclusion	**Induction always works**

The outcome of Hume's deliberations is to remove any certainty concerning the results of inductive reasoning. If there is no sound basis for induction, then any argument from observation instances to a generalisation remains open to question. In other words, Hume's stance was one of extreme scepticism with regard to induction. But, while holding firmly to his philosophical analysis, he was fully aware of the central role that induction plays in our lives and recognised the impossibility of simply dismissing inductive reasoning on the grounds that it was unproven. And, as when faced with conflicts between the outcome of philosophical analysis and our lives in the natural world, Hume reverted to a naturalistic position: *"... nature has not left this to our choice and has doubtless esteemed it an affair of too great importance to be trusted to our uncertain reasonings and speculations...That is a point which we must take for granted in all our reasonings."* [5]

By our nature, we think according to the principle of induction and we behave as if such inferences were reliable. Despite the absence of a firm intellectual foundation for inductive inference, we still make generalisations based on observation instances and we continue to rely on these generalisations. And, of course, we have little choice in the matter. Without our actions being guided by inductive inference, we could not build shelter from the elements or make fires, we could not collect water or grow food. Our nature is such that we believe that what happens in the future will resemble the past. Induction permeates all our lives. There is no escape from it. We may accept Hume's sceptical account and question the insubstantial basis for induction but, if we are to survive, we must act as if the future will resemble the past and as if observation instances from the past provide support for generalisations which may reliably be projected into the future.

Hume

- **Induction is not logically necessary**

- **Arguments based on the principle of induction working successfully in the past are circular**

- **We have a natural disposition to believe in induction**

However, while a naturalistic account may describe a phenomenon - in this case, our natural disposition to embrace inductive thinking - it does not provide an argument demonstrating the validity of such inferences. Hume's critique of induction, therefore, remains an obstacle to any claim for certainty in the outcome of inductive inference. But, although it is possible that any particular inductive generalisation may prove to be false, many such generalisations have been shown to be reliable over long periods of time and are as certain as any items of knowledge. All animals need oxygen to stay alive, ice is cold, granite slabs do not float in water, lemons are sour tasting - these are universally accepted generalisations and anyone claiming the contrary would be viewed with the utmost suspicion. Despite Hume's insights, we maintain confidence in such generalisations.

Causation

Causation may be considered as part of the more general notion of induction. A series of observation instances may provide support for either non-causal generalisations – for example, "all monkeys have lungs" or "solutions of copper sulphate are blue" – or causal generalisations such as "all lions die if deprived of oxygen" or "ice melts if warmed above $0°C$". Causal generalisations involve a particular kind of relationship between objects or events. In other words, they describe a causal link between, for example, raising the temperature above $0°C$ and the melting of ice.

While the notion of causation is complex, we use causal concepts as a matter routine in our everyday lives. Their complexity does not trouble us because we have learned their intricacies along with the rest of language. We develop expertise in the field of causal reasoning. And, as a result, we are able to use these concepts for a wide variety of practical purposes. Consider the causal generalisation "wax candles melt when in contact with a flame". Everyone understands this statement and few would disagree with it. But how do we know that this generalisation is true? The answer is that our experiences support this conclusion. From pictures in children's books of molten wax running down the sides of burning candles and films of Ebenezer Scrooge counting his money by candlelight, to our own direct experiences - at birthday parties, in church, when the electricity fails, at Hallowe'en and Christmas time - we learn about the behaviour of wax candles. All our experiences record a regular association between the flame and the melting of the candle. However, the inference from past instances to the generalisation that "wax candles melt when in contact with a flame" is not made in a vacuum. We have knowledge of similar phenomena. Other objects melt when exposed to heat – butter in a warm saucepan, chocolate left in direct sunlight, tarmac on the roads during a heat-wave and solder touched with a hot iron. Such phenomena provide a background against which the generalisation concerning wax candles may be interpreted. Given that other objects melt when exposed to heat, it is not unreasonable to accept that wax candles behave in the same way. Without any conscious use of induction, we learn this reliable generalisation and use it for practical purposes. We know that candles melt when in contact with a flame, so much so that were the opposite to occur we would not accept the observation statement at face value.

However, although we have no difficulty in using causal language in everyday matters, problems arise when we try to analyse the concept of causation. What, for instance, constitutes a causal relationship? And how is such a relationship recognised? What conditions must be satisfied before we are entitled to assert that one object or event causes another? Given the central importance of causation to science, these questions have to be addressed.

It is rare to encounter any serious exposition of causation that does not include reference to David Hume. As with induction, his insights into causation remain paramount in the literature. Hume sought to determine the precise nature of causal relationships. He, of course, accepted that a cause precedes its effect and that they are located in close proximity. Apart from these two features, however, he was unable to identify any other factor involved in the perception of an instance of causation. *"Having thus discover'd or suppos'd the two relations of contiguity and succession to be essential to causes and effects, I find I am stopt short, and can proceed no farther in considering any single instance of cause and effect."* [6] Thus, as far as perception is concerned, there is nothing else to a causal relationship except temporal priority and spatial proximity.

Having rejected perception as providing a satisfactory account of causation, Hume proceeded to attack the idea that the causal connection is based on logic, in other words, that a cause logically entails its effect. If we take any situation in the natural world, we can imagine a particular cause not being followed by its effect; if we can imagine a situation, then it is logically possible; but, if it is logically possible that the cause is not followed by its effect, then it cannot be the case that the relationship between a cause and its effect is based on logical necessity.

In *An Essay Concerning Human Understanding* (1689), John Locke offered an account of causation which focussed on the way in which a cause is involved in the production of its effect: *"a cause is that which makes any other thing... begin to be, and an effect is that which has its beginning from some other thing..."* [7] Thus, a cause is not merely associated in space and time with the effect but it brings about its effect. Hume, though, was dismissive of this generative theory of causation: *"Shou'd any one... pretend to define a cause, by saying it is something productive of another, 'tis evident he wou'd say nothing... Can he give a definition of [production], that will not be the same with that of causation ? If he can; I desire it may be produc'd. If he cannot; he here runs in a circle."* [8] While the generative theory is entirely in keeping with our everyday understanding of causation, Hume's argument is that the theory cannot be used to explain the origin of the connection between a cause and its effect without circularity.

As with induction, Hume's enquiries seem to have destroyed any possibility that causal relationships may be founded on logic or experience. But, as with induction, when faced with stark scepticism concerning a fundamental feature of our lives, he turned to naturalism. Our belief in the causal relationship stems from a natural disposition: *"We remember to have had frequent instances of the existence of one species of objects; and also remember, that the individuals of another species of objects have always attended them, and have existed in a regular order of contiguity and succession with regard to them... Without any farther ceremony, we call the one cause and the other effect, and infer the existence of the one from that of the other."* [9] In terms of what we actually perceive, there is nothing more to causation than two objects or events associated in space and time; but it is the repetition of similar observations that produces the ideas of cause and effect.

Our belief in causation is the result of a natural disposition and this belief is strengthened as the number of instances which we observe increases: *"The first instance has little or no force: The second makes some addition to it: The third becomes still more sensible; and 'tis by these slow steps, that our judgment arrives at a full assurance...".* [10] But, in the absence of firm foundations for causation, Hume's "full assurance" has rather half-hearted undertones and his scepticism is seldom far below the surface: *"Twou'd be very happy for men in the conduct of their lives and actions, were the same objects always conjoin'd together, and we had nothing to fear but the mistakes of our own judgment, without having any reason to apprehend the uncertainty of nature."* [11]

This last quotation is of interest because it anticipates the practical problems involved with the identification of cause and effect relationships. As always, Hume was acutely aware of the nature of these difficulties and issued a warning: *"... all kinds of reasoning from causes to effects are founded on two particulars, viz. the constant conjunction of any two objects in all past experience, and the resemblance of a present object to any one of them... If you weaken either the union or resemblance, you weaken the principle of transition, and of consequence that belief, which arises from it."* [12] The importance of this quotation, to science in general and medicine in particular, cannot be overemphasized. It stipulates the conditions necessary for reliable causal generalisations, namely the requirement that the generalisation is based on consistent observations of the association between the supposed cause and its effect with no conflicting observation instances, and the requirement that the items involved in the generalisation belong to homogeneous classes. Whenever these conditions are not met, the reliability of any causal inference is brought into question.

Hume provided two definitions of causation. The first is a philosophical definition of a cause: *"'An object precedent and contiguous to another, and where all the objects resembling the former are plac'd in like relations of priority and contiguity to those objects, that resemble the latter."* [13] This specifies the conditions required in order for a causal relationship to be established and provides the basis for what has become known as the regularity theory of causation. The second is a psychological definition of a cause: *"An object precedent and contiguous to another, and so united with it, that the idea of one determines the mind to form the idea of the other…"*. [13] This emphasizes that the origin of our belief in causation lies in our natural disposition to interpret repeated associations in this manner. The second definition also draws attention to Hume's view that causation is not something that exists in the world apart from a regular association but rather is a construction of the human mind.

Hume's Regularity Theory of Causation

- **Temporal priority**
- **Spatial contiguity**
- **Resemblance**
- **Repetition of patterns**

It is interesting to note that Hume drew attention to the complex nature of causal relationships and proposed a method of approaching this problem: *"There is no phenomenon in nature, but what is compounded and modify'd by so many different circumstances, that in order to arrive at the decisive point, we must carefully separate whatever is superfluous, and enquire by new experiments, if every particular circumstance of the first experiment was essential to it. These new experiments are liable to a discussion of the same kind..."* [14] The suggestion appears to be that the circumstances surrounding a particular case of a causal relationship should be analysed by isolating the various components in order to assess their relevance; having identified the relevant factors, a series of experiments would then be performed to determine their role in causation.

Hume was not the first philosopher to describe the regularity theory. Thomas Hobbes provided an early account in *Leviathan* (1651)[15] as did John Locke in *An Essay Concerning Human Understanding* (1689).[7] However, Hume's unique contributions were decisive in ensuring that the regularity theory would remain central to causation. In *A System of Logic* (1843), JS Mill provided a detailed and pragmatic exposition of induction and causation which openly supported the regularity theory: *"To certain facts, certain other facts always do, and, as we believe, will continue to, succeed. The invariable antecedent is termed the cause; the invariable consequent, the effect."* [16] The regularity theory survived throughout the twentieth century as shown, for example, in JL Mackie's *The Cement of the Universe* (1974)[17]. Indeed, the title of this work - perhaps the most comprehensive account of causation since the Second World War - was taken directly from David Hume.

In summary, induction and causation are central to our understanding of the natural world. Without causal inference, purposeful action would not be possible and we would be unable to manipulate the environment to our advantage. Causation, too, is central to science. The aim of all experiments is to identify causal relationships, all experiments involve causal inference and all yield causal generalisations. Hence, an understanding of causation - of what it means and how it is established - is of the utmost importance for any appreciation of the scientific method.

The Scientific Method

In contrast to everyday situations, science relates to phenomena that are often obscure and unfamiliar to us. As a result, the informal processes that usually combine to produce reliable generalisations from our experiences are no longer suitable; something more is needed. To compensate for the absence of the usual mechanisms that protect against insecure generalisations, science has had to introduce a formal structure to the process of induction.

Any account of the scientific method is incomplete without mention of Francis Bacon. In his major works - *Advancement of Learning (1605)* and *Novum Organum (1620)*[18] - he described the fundamental principles of scientific investigation. He was critical of the view, prevalent at the time, that knowledge was acquired from reasoning alone and instead emphasized the crucial importance of empirical experience. He proposed that the search for knowledge should begin with observations from which, over time, generalisations would be derived. But in order for generalisations to be reliable, Bacon realised that account must be taken of the occurrence of any negative instance, that is, an observation that conflicts with the generalisation. Whilst this may seem all too obvious, he drew attention to our inclination to ignore such observations: *"...it is the peculiar and perpetual error of human intellect to be more moved and excited by affirmatives than by negatives."*.[19] This bias remains endemic four centuries after Bacon's pronouncements and is evident not only in the case of the inveterate gambler who recalls only those occasions when he has left the racecourse with his wallet bulging with notes, but also in medical science, where generalisations based on the results of a number of studies are accepted in the face of contradictory evidence from other trials.

Bacon's Insights

- **Scientific knowledge begins with observations of particular instances which yield generalisations**

- **The importance of the negative instance**

- **Systematic experiment with varying conditions to identify factors involved in the phenomenon (variative induction)**

Perhaps, though, Bacon's greatest contribution to science was his insistence on the experimental method. He was dismissive of induction which relied solely on the number of observations made and favoured instead the identification and manipulation of those factors involved in any phenomenon: *"...induction which proceeds by simple enumeration is childish; its conclusions are precarious, and exposed to peril from a contradictory instance... But the induction which is to be available for the discovery and demonstration of sciences must analyse nature by proper rejections and exclusions"*.[20] There is a fundamental difference between these two approaches to induction. Enumerative induction focuses attention on to the number of instances without any concern given to the observations being carried out under different conditions. Variative induction, on the other hand, is a method of reaching a generalisation where the validity of the generalisation has been tested over a wide variety of different conditions. If the variation in conditions shows that the generalisation does not hold, then it must be rejected or modified.

These three insights - that scientific knowledge should be based on empirical experience, that negative instances must not be ignored and that variative, rather than enumerative, induction is the foundation of the scientific method - justify Bacon's pivotal role in the development of modern science.

Factors affecting the reliability of scientific generalisations

A simplified version of the conditions required for reliable generalisations in science is often presented as follows: if a large number of instances of X have been observed over a wide variety of conditions and every instance of X has shown characteristic Y without exception, then we may infer "all X's are Y". This statement, though, while summarising some of the important features of a successful approach to inductive inference, is too simplistic and requires modification.

Induction

Observation of → **Generalisations**
particular instances

Reliability depends on:
- **Background theory**
- **Reference class description**
- **Number of observations**
- **Variety of conditions**
- **No conflicting observations**

Observations are dependent on theory

The act of observation may appear to be simple but it is a very complex activity. The rays of light that leave an abstract picture on the wall of the art gallery and pass through the cornea before striking the retinae of two individuals are the same, but the picture reported by each is different. Similarly, the sound waves from the violin that pass through the air and vibrate the tympanic membrane are the same but the description of what is heard may be different. The differences arise from the fact that when the sensory organs project the neural signals to the higher centres, the brain processes the information. This processing is performed against a background of previous experience, knowledge, theories, expectations and cultural attitudes.

Consider the following example of a medical student asked to auscultate a patient's heart. He listens attentively before reporting the breath sounds from the lungs, the first and second heart sounds and extraneous noises from the contact between the stethoscope and the chest wall. The cardiologist then repeats the exercise, confirming all the findings of the medical student but, in addition, reporting an early diastolic murmur at the left sternal edge. In this case, the sounds presented to the tympanic membranes of the medical student and the cardiologist are the same but the interpretation is different. The cardiologist is accustomed to listening to the various phases of the cardiac cycle separately; he is able to focus his attention individually on the first sound, the second sound, systole, diastole and any added sounds; he is attuned to the sound of early diastolic murmurs - he has heard them thousands of times before. In contrast, the medical student has no such expertise and the early diastolic murmur passes unnoticed. As this case demonstrates, observations are influenced by previous knowledge and experience.

> **Observations are never simple**
>
> **Observation depends on:**
> - **Previous experience**
> - **Knowledge**
> - **Expectations**
> - **Pre-existing theory**

Observations, however, are also made against a background of pre-existing theory. Consider the following observation statement: "after being exposed to oxygen and water, this piece of iron is covered in rust". How does the person reporting the observation know that it is a piece of iron and not some other metal? There are many possible replies: "it was produced from iron ore by a specific process.... it has a relative density of 7.87.... it has a melting point of 1535^0C.... it reacts with hydrochloric acid to produce...." All these features, however, refer back to established generalisations, for example, "iron melts at 1535^0C". And the same applies to the other terms - 'oxygen', 'water' and 'rust' - involved in the observation statement. Hence, observation statements are dependent upon pre-existing theory. As Karl Popper stated unequivocally: *"...the belief that we can start with pure observations alone, without a theory, is absurd... observation is always selective... observation statements are always interpretations of the facts observed... interpretations in the light of theories."* [21]

These considerations bring into question the reliability of observations. In particular, while the physical sciences are characterised by sound background theory and knowledge which deliver precise definitions, this is not the case in other disciplines, especially medical research.

Resemblance between observation instances

It is self-evident that inductive inference relies upon the similarity between the items of each observation instance. The generalisation "all X's are Y" implies that each instance of X resembles the other instances in terms of those characteristics which define X.

A generalisation such as "all cats chase mice" is based on a series of observations each of which report an instance of a particular cat chasing a mouse. Behind this inference lies the notion of analogy: if these animals with four legs, nine lives, whiskers, pointed ears, a fondness for drinking milk chase mice, then this animal with the same characteristics will also chase mice. Analogy, however, not only depends on similarities but also on differences. If a particular cat had features different from other cats - for example, it was paralysed or under the influence of a sedative drug - then the inappropriateness of the analogy would be readily apparent. A further aspect of reasoning by analogy is the importance of the relevance of the features. For example, the colour of the cat or the length of its tail would be considered irrelevant to the generalisation that "all cats chase mice" because such features would not be expected to affect the natural inclination of these animals to chase mice. Clearly, though, the identification of relevant as opposed to irrelevant features is dependent upon background knowledge and pre-existing theory.

In the physical sciences, the definitions of objects involved in a generalisation are usually precise and unambiguous. For example, in the generalisation "iron exposed to water and oxygen produces rust", there is no debate about the definitions of iron, water, oxygen or rust. If a particular piece of metal satisfies the criteria by which iron is defined and is exposed to both oxygen and water for a specified period of time, rust will develop. The reliability of generalisations in the physical sciences is founded on the precision of the definitions used. This, of course, is not to claim either that the conditions of each observation instance that yield the generalisation are identical or that future instances must be identical to those from which the generalisation was derived. Despite the paramount concern in science with accurate measurement, no two pieces of iron are absolutely identical - they do not, for example, contain precisely the same number of atoms, they are located in different places, etc. But, in those respects that are relevant to the generalisation under consideration, the subtle differences that are present do not affect the outcome to any practical extent. It is in this sense, then, that the items involved in the statements of the physical sciences may be said to be homogeneous.

It is a strict requirement of science that the terms used in observation statements and generalisations refer to items that are as homogeneous as possible. However, the degree to which items need to resemble one another - in other words the degree of homogeneity - depends on the context. If the generalisation concerned the melting point of metals, the shape and size would be less relevant than in the context of ballistics.

Homogeneous Classes

- **Differences between items involved in the observations are not relevant to the generalisation**

- **Crucial requirement of the scientific method**

- **Readily satisfied in the physical sciences**

Away form the clarity of the physical sciences, definitions become vague and hence the resemblance between observation instances lessens. In no sphere of science is this problem more evident than in medicine. The basic building blocks of observation statements leading to generalisations in medicine include 'patients', 'symptoms', 'signs', 'diagnosis', and 'treatment'. These terms, however, are imprecise. Each patient has their own specific identity which is the result of a constellation of characteristics: they are of different heights and weights, and the dimensions of their hearts, lungs and livers vary widely; the colour of their skin, eyes and hair is different, as is their blood group and tissue type; they have different voices, run at different speeds, have different resting heart rates, different lung volumes, and different rates of absorption, metabolism and excretion; they have different personalities, different intellects; and, excluding monozygotic twins, they all have a different genetic make-up. Given these differences, 'patients' usually refers to a heterogeneous class of individuals.

In certain circumstances, the term 'patients' may comprise a homogeneous class: "all patients have a brain" and "all patients will die if deprived of oxygen" are reliable, if crude, generalisations. However, in most instances, the differences among individual human beings - whether in terms of their normal anatomical, physiological or biochemical characteristics, or in terms of their pathology - are relevant to the proposed generalisation. Outside of the sphere of the physical sciences, and especially in medicine, the requirement for homogeneous classes is seldom fulfilled although the degree of heterogeneity present will vary in different contexts.

Induction in the physical sciences leads to very accurate predictions about the future and much of this success is related to the isolation of homogeneous classes of objects involved in the generalisations. In contrast, medical science has no such ready access to homogeneous classes and, as a result, the reliability of the generalisations is greatly lessened.

Enumerative versus variative induction

Enumerative induction favours the number - as opposed to the variety - of observation instances that form the basis of a generalisation. If a large number of observations have been made and each of these instances reports that X has feature Y, then, in line with enumerative induction, the evidence supports the generalisation "all X's have feature Y". Before the late 18th Century, millions of observations from all over England, from the rest of Europe and elsewhere in the northern hemisphere reported that swans were white. On the basis of this vast amount of evidence, it would appear reasonable to infer that "all swans are white". But, despite the huge number of instances, this inference proved to be unreliable when black swans were discovered in Western Australia. Again, imagine that a very large number of observations showed that pure water boils at 100°C but that all of these observations had taken place at or near sea-level. On the basis that the reliability of inductive inference increases with a large number of observations, the generalisation "all pure water boils at 100°C" would appear justified. However, the visitor in a hotel in Quito or the mountaineer in a tent at the foothills of Mount Everest would clearly be able to contest the claim. Bacon was correct when he criticised enumerative induction; it is demonstrably inadequate for the formation of reliable conclusions because, by its very nature, it does not formally address the variety of conditions that ultimately may falsify the generalisation. In the case of the boiling point of water, for example, the generalisation was unwarranted because the effects of a crucially relevant factor, *viz.* atmospheric pressure, were not taken into consideration.

The fundamental feature of variative induction - often referred to as "Baconian induction" - is that observations are performed under different conditions which bring to light factors which potentially challenge the reliability of a generalisation. These factors are known as relevant variables because their presence affects the outcome in question. For example, atmospheric pressure is a relevant variable for the boiling point of water and if it is not taken into consideration, any resulting generalisation such as "all pure water boils at 100°C" will simply be false.

The effect of relevant variables is studied either by further observations under naturally occurring different conditions or by deliberate manipulation of the conditions in a formal experiment. In the case of the boiling point of water, the effect of atmospheric pressure would be identified either by measurements taken at various altitudes or by varying the pressure in an experimental situation. In either case, the results would show that atmospheric pressure is a relevant variable and that the generalisation "all pure water boils at 100°C" requires modification - for example, "all pure water boils at 100°C at sea-level in containers open to the atmosphere" - if it is to apply universally.

Variative induction is the primary process by which false generalisations are avoided. However, it must be recognised that the assessment of the effects of relevant variables requires their recognition which, in turn, depends on background knowledge and theory. Moreover, whatever the level of knowledge, it remains possible that other unknown relevant variables may weaken a generalisation.

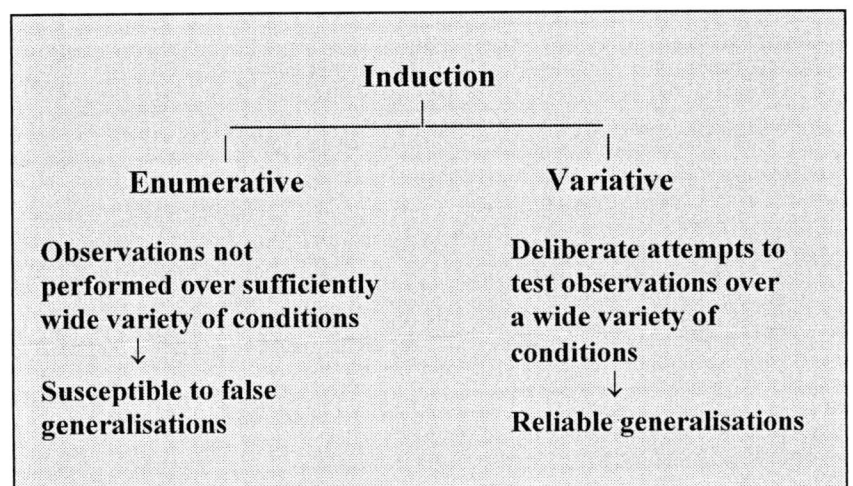

Negative instances

In the physical sciences, an observation instance which conflicts with a generalisation is subjected to rigorous investigation in order to determine differences between the initial conditions of the negative instance and those which support the generalisation. The outcome may be the rejection of the observation statement, the rejection of the generalisation or the modification of the generalisation if a new relevant variable were to be identified. This attention to the negative instance allows science to deliver universal generalisations. For example, the statement "copper expands when heated" applies to all samples of that metal without exception.

In medicine, on the other hand, generalisations are rarely universal; instead, they are particular statements which attribute a characteristic only to a proportion of the reference class. "Beta-blockers reduce mortality from ischaemic heart disease" is a composite of two different statements – "beta-blockers prevent death in some patients" and "beta-blockers do not prevent death in some patients". In this way, negative instances are accommodated. It is in the nature of the subject matter of much of medical research that universal generalisations are not possible and negative instances remain unchallenged.

Negative Instance	
Physical sciences	**Medicine**
Question validity of observation statement or reject or modify the generalisation	Negative instances accepted unchallenged

The relevance of the negative instance is that it raises a fundamental objection to the generalisation under consideration. Of course, an observation statement that conflicts with the generalisation may itself be questioned but, if it cannot be rejected, then the generalisation itself must be rejected. The failure to take due account of the negative instances in medicine reduces the reliability of the generalisations and encourages the inclusion of contradictory statements which threatens the entire body of knowledge.

Replication
Science involves precise definition of the materials and methods which, amongst other things, enables the experiment to be repeated under exactly the same conditions. Replication is an essential feature of the scientific method and is the primary means by which investigators verify the results of published studies. This does not mean that every experiment is immediately subjected to verification. Usually, an unexpected result will prompt attempts to repeat the experiment. Alternatively, efforts to replicate the original findings may also follow conflicting results from other studies of similar phenomena. But, irrespective of the source, the failure to

replicate the findings of a scientific experiment casts serious doubt on the initial results and prevents their incorporation into the body of scientific knowledge.

In the context of medical research, the failure to specify accurately the characteristics of the patients and their diseases prevents any firm attempt at replication. Thus, clinical trials may be criticised on the grounds that they do not comply with this fundamental aspect of the scientific method.

Scientific theories and paradigms

The scientific process leads to the formation of broad theories that provide explanations for a wide range of phenomena which we observe in the world. Isaac Newton's theory, which dominated science for more than 200 years, is a prime example of a theory with broad scope. His laws of motion and gravity unified a vast number of diverse phenomena from the results of experiments in the laboratory to the movements of the planets. Newton's theory obeys the requirements of all successful theories: it provides a framework for thinking about the workings of nature and allows accurate predictions of future events.

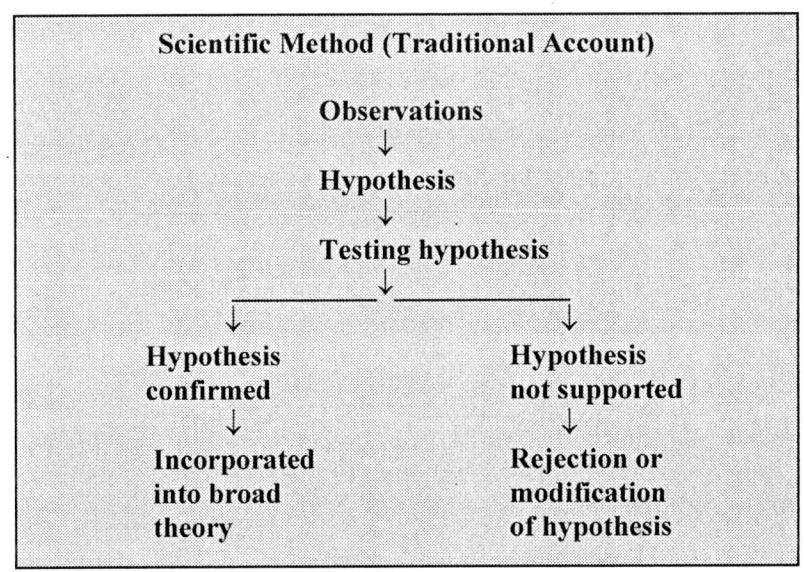

The traditional account of the scientific process begins with observations. From observations are derived generalisations which, because they require confirmation, are referred to as hypotheses. Each hypothesis is subjected to tests which involve the manipulation of relevant variables; the hypothesis is then either confirmed or rejected. Those hypotheses which are confirmed are then incorporated into a theory from which further hypotheses are derived and subsequently tested in a similar manner. Finally, a broad theory is derived which has wide application to many diverse phenomena in the world.

From this perspective, it would seem as though theory was solely the end product of the scientific process. This view, however, ignores the function of theory in the earlier stages of the process; the importance of this contribution cannot be overstated. Theory is involved in the identification and selection of observation statements; it plays a role in the interpretation of these statements and the subsequent development of hypotheses; it is of crucial importance in the design of experiments, particularly in respect of the selection of relevant variables to be examined, and in the interpretation of the results; and the theory provides a framework for the acceptance or rejection of new findings.

In one of the most influential works on the philosophy of science published since the Second World War, *The Structure of Scientific Revolutions* [1962],[22] Thomas Kuhn introduced the concept of a paradigm. At the centre of this work is the idea that each science is practiced within a single paradigm which consists of, among other things, basic theory, fundamental laws and essential methodology. The paradigm provides guidance for the investigation and advancement of theories. It is a framework, a background to the practice of science. According to Kuhn, science progresses through stages: 'normal science' is a problem-solving activity, the aim of which is to improve the agreement between nature and the paradigm; over time, problems arise in the form of new evidence which accumulates to the point of threatening the paradigm and eventually a crisis develops in which the paradigm itself is doubted; a rival paradigm emerges which fits the evidence better than its predecessor; finally, a scientific revolution occurs and the new paradigm prevails; a new 'normal science' has arrived. Kuhn's ideas are most readily applicable to the established sciences, in particular physics and chemistry. But in other disciplines - for example, psychology, psychiatry and sociology - the notion of a paradigm appears unsuitable.

Medicine is clearly not governed by a single paradigm. It involves contributions from a wide spectrum of disciplines ranging from those governed by a single paradigm to those still in search of a broad, fundamental theory. The absence of a paradigm in medicine is important. Without a background of strong theory and knowledge, the scientific process is weakened: definitions are vague, identification of relevant variables is limited and there is no framework against which to judge the outcome of experiments. Medical science comprises a large number of generalisations that tend to exist independently without any supporting structure. Hypotheses that have seemingly been confirmed are accepted piecemeal, including conflicting evidence. Rudimentary 'theories' abound, survive briefly and are then abandoned, only to be replaced by yet more rudimentary theories.

Conclusions

Induction is an integral part of human life. It lies behind our everyday actions and without at the very least a tacit acceptance of induction purposeful action would not be possible. Whilst agreeing with Hume's philosophical arguments that we cannot prove its validity, we must accept that induction yields reliable generalisations on which we may base our decisions. Put simply, we have no alternative but to act in accordance with induction and causation.

In our everyday lives, we have little difficulty in using the concepts of induction and causation, and we do not doubt that most of the generalisations derived from these inferences are secure. We *know*, for instance, that all human beings have a heart and lungs inside their chest. And we *know* that a stone dropped from a height will fall to the ground. The objects involved in such statements are extremely familiar to us and the generalisations are connected with many other things of which we are certain, so much so that were we to question their validity, we would also be questioning many other areas of knowledge.

Science is founded on the principles of induction and causation. Although the phenomena under investigation are often unfamiliar and even obscure, sound background theory and knowledge ensure precise definitions of the components of an experiment. The scientific method centres on the construction of experiments involving homogeneous reference classes and the manipulation of relevant variables, conditions which deliver universal generalisations. The importance of background theory and knowledge in relation to observation, the formation of hypotheses, the design of experiments to test hypotheses and the interpretation of the results is clear. The reliability of generalisations in science depends not only on the results of a particular set of observations but also on the way in which a generalisation is supported within a wider framework of experimental evidence and theory.

As Hume argued, the identification of a causal relationship depends on the conditions of the regularity theory. It is a fundamental characteristic of the scientific method that it attempts to create these conditions. For causal generalisations to be reliable, there must be a regular association between two sets of objects or events where the objects or events in each set resemble one another sufficiently closely to be classified as homogeneous. The experiments of science, which seek to identify causal relationships, comply with these requirements and, in consequence, are able to deliver reliable generalisations.

But, whenever the circumstances deviate from regularity and resemblance, the validity of causal inference is brought into question. This is the situation which nowadays faces those involved in much of clinical research.

References

1. Hume D. *A Treatise of Human Nature (1739)*. Edited by EC Mossner. Penguin Books Ltd, Middlesex, England, 1987.

2. Hume D. *Enquiries concerning Human Understanding and concerning the Principles of Morals (1777)*. Edited by LA Selby-Bigge. Clarendon Press, Oxford, 1983.

3. Hume D. *A Treatise of Human Nature (1739)*. Edited by EC Mossner. Penguin Books Ltd, Middlesex, England, 1987. Bk I; Pt III; Sect VI; P137.

4. Hume D. *An Enquiry concerning Human Understanding (1777)*. Edited by LA Selby-Bigge. Clarendon Press, Oxford, 1983. Bk I, Part II, Sect IV, P37-38.

5. Hume D. *A Treatise of Human Nature (1739)*. Edited by EC Mossner. Penguin Books Ltd, Middlesex, England, 1987. Bk I, Part IV, Sect II, P238.

6. Hume D. *A Treatise of Human Nature (1739)*. Edited by EC Mossner. Penguin Books Ltd, Middlesex, England, 1987. Bk I; Part III; Section II; P124.

7. Locke J. *An Essay concerning Human Understanding (1689)*. Abridged and edited by JW Yolton. Guernsey Press Co. Ltd. 1976. Bk II; Cap XXVI; P155.

8. Hume D. *A Treatise of Human Nature (1739)*. Edited by EC Mossner. Penguin Books Ltd, Middlesex, England, 1987. Bk I; Part III; Section II; P124-125.

9. Hume D. *A Treatise of Human Nature (1739)*. Edited by EC Mossner. Penguin Books Ltd, Middlesex, England, 1987. Bk I; Part III; Sect VI; P135.

10. Hume D. *A Treatise of Human Nature (1739)*. Edited by EC Mossner. Penguin Books Ltd, Middlesex, England, 1987. Bk I; Part III; Sect XII; P181.

11. Hume D. *A Treatise of Human Nature (1739)*. Edited by EC Mossner. Penguin Books Ltd, Middlesex, England, 1987. Bk I; Part III; Sect XII; P182.

12. Hume D. *A Treatise of Human Nature (1739)*. Edited by EC Mossner. Penguin Books Ltd, Middlesex, England, 1987. Bk I; Part III; Sect XII; P192.

13. Hume D. *A Treatise of Human Nature (1739)*. Edited by EC Mossner. Penguin Books Ltd, Middlesex, England, 1987. Bk I; Part III; Sect XIV; P222.

14. Hume D. *A Treatise of Human Nature (1739)*. Edited by EC Mossner. Penguin Books Ltd, Middlesex, England, 1987. Bk I; Part III; Sect XV; P225.

15. Hobbes T. *Leviathan (1651)*. Edited by J Plamenatz; William Collins Sons & Co. Ltd, Glasgow, 1962.

16. Mill JS. *A System of Logic*. Longmans, Green & Co. London, 1884. Bk III; Chap V; Sect 2; P213.

17. Mackie JL. *The Cement of the Universe*. Oxford University Press. Oxford, 1974.

18. Bacon F. *Works*. Edited by J Spedding, RL Ellis and DD Heath. London. 1857-74.

19. Bacon F. *Works*. Edited by J Spedding, RL Ellis and DD Heath. London. 1857-74. *First Book of Aphorisms*. XLVI.

20. Bacon F. *Works*. Edited by J Spedding, RL Ellis and DD Heath. London. 1857-74. *First Book of Aphorisms*. CV.

21. Popper K. *The Logic of Scientific Discovery*. Hutchinson, 1959.

22. Kuhn T. *The Structure of Scientific Revolutions.* University of Chicago Press; Chicago, 1962.

III

RANDOMISATION - A CLEVER MOVE
OR AN ACT OF DESPERATION?

The development of safe and effective general anaesthetics, the improvements in surgical techniques, organ transplantation, insulin and other hormone replacement therapies, antibiotics.... the list of advances in medicine during the past hundred years is both long and impressive. However, many diseases – in particular, those responsible for most of the morbidity and mortality in developed countries – have proved resistant to the efforts of medical researchers. This is because much of medicine is hampered by the vagueness of its subject matter and by its lack of a solid theoretical structure to guide observations, to select homogeneous classes, to assist with the identification of relevant variables and to process the results of studies. The clarity characteristic of science is lacking and, instead, medical researchers are faced with highly complex situations.

In *A System of Logic* (1843), JS Mill commented graphically on this complexity: *"The order of nature, as perceived at a first glance, presents at every instant a chaos followed by another chaos... We must learn to see in the chaotic antecedent a multitude of distinct antecedents, in the chaotic consequent a multitude of distinct consequents... we must endeavour to effect a separation of the facts from one another, not only in our minds but in nature."* [1] While his approach to the identification of causal relationships has been criticised, his emphasis on the clear recognition and isolation of the factors involved as pre-requisites for the establishment of causation by means of experiments is worthy of note.[2] The medical research community, though, has failed to take account of Mill's advice. Confronted by the problem of how to derive reliable generalisations from the endemic chaos created by the innumerable differences among patients, the standard scientific method has been judged unsuitable and, instead, an alternative methodology has been developed, namely, the randomised controlled trial. On the surface, it bears all the hallmarks of scientific respectability; but, on closer inspection, its weaknesses are brought into focus.

History of the Randomised Clinical Trial

In 1898, Johannes Fibiger published the results of a study of the treatment of diphtheria which nowadays is regarded as the earliest example of the randomised controlled clinic trial.[3] His insight was to recognise the requirement for some mechanism to ensure that the two treatment groups were evenly matched: *"...the control cases... selected to be as similar as possible to the ones treated with the serum, but to eliminate completely the play of chance and the influence of subjective judgment..."* [4] Fibiger's chosen method was for alternate day allocation to either serum treatment or no active treatment: *"The only method which could be used rationally was to treat some patients with serum and every other patient in the usual way"*.

It was not until the 1930's that further attempts at randomisation were made in medicine: the toss of a coin was used to allocate patients with tuberculosis to treatment with gold[5] while alternate allocation to active treatment was used in patients with pneumonia[6] and the common cold.[7] The first randomised controlled clinical trial began in 1946, although it did not appear in print until 1951, and involved pertussis immunisation.[8] The first published randomised controlled trial[9], reporting the treatment of tuberculosis with streptomycin, appeared in 1948 and issued in a new era of clinical research which, during the ensuing fifty years, included the publication of more than half a million randomised trials.

The Need for Randomisation

The aim of any clinical trial is to detect a difference in the specified outcome between two or more groups and to attribute this to a difference in treatment. In other words, the fundamental objective of clinical trials is the identification of causal relationships. However, in order to ensure that any difference in outcome is related to the difference in exposure or treatment, the groups must be matched in all other respects.

Individual human beings differ from one another in an almost infinite number of respects – from their physical dimensions to the number of parietal cells in their stomach, from the amount of cytochrome P450 in their liver to their creatinine clearance, and from their psychological profile to their genetic make-up, to name but a few. And each disease affects individuals in different ways and to a variable extent. Some of these differences will be recognised to affect the outcome of a clinical trial, others may be suspected of doing so while, of the vast majority, little will be known. Thus, any study population will comprise a group of individuals who vary in terms of factors which potentially affect the outcome under investigation. Even if it were theoretically possible for our knowledge to extend to every minute detail of every factor relevant to the outcome of the disease, it would, in practical terms, be impossible to create two treatment groups matched in every respect. As a consequence, any claim that a difference in outcome of a clinical trial between one group and another is due to the effect of treatment may be challenged on the grounds that the difference may reflect an unequal distribution of other relevant variables.

Faced with this seemingly intractable problem, clinical researchers in the 1940's seized upon the mechanism of randomisation. As Austin Bradford Hill stated, the purpose of randomisation is *"...to ensure beforehand that, as far as possible, the control and the treated groups are the same in all relevant respects"* [10] In such circumstances, knowledge of the relevant variables is assumed to be unnecessary because all of these – whether known or unknown – are believed to be distributed equally amongst the different groups and hence differences in outcome may be attributed to differences in treatment alone. In practice, however, the randomisation process struggles to achieve its aim of equally matched groups.

Problems with Randomisation

The initial phase of randomisation

(i) The randomisation process, by definition, entails the generation of a sequence entirely on the basis of chance, yet claims that treatment is allocated randomly are not always justified. Unless the method is accurately specified, the possibility that a non-random process has been used must be considered.[11] Unfortunately, assessment of the extent of this problem is hampered by the frequent failure of publications to describe the method of sequence generation.

(ii) Investigators responsible for the recruitment of patients must remain ignorant of the next treatment delivered by the randomisation process until patients have been formally assigned to that treatment. Interference with random allocation so that particular patients are preferentially assigned to one treatment group leads to selection bias.[12,13] The omission of a description of allocation concealment from publications is not uncommon and should be viewed with suspicion. Furthermore, there is ample evidence in the literature of researchers subverting the process of allocation concealment [12-14] although the scale of the problem – as with research misconduct in general – is unknown. Currently, the preferred method of concealment is for clinical researchers to contact a randomisation centre by telephone and provide details of the patient before the allocation of treatment is issued. [12,13]

(iii) Much attention has been given to baseline imbalance, in other words, the formation of groups which are unequal in terms of either the number of patients or the distribution of relevant variables.[14-16] Baseline imbalance may arise from the randomisation process simply due to chance; although this is predominantly a feature of smaller trials, it is worth noting that minor degrees of baseline imbalance may be of importance in large-scale trials where the treatment difference is always small. For example, the conclusions of recent multi-centre randomised trials – the HOPE study[17] and the LIFE study[18] - have been challenged on the grounds of baseline imbalance.[19,20] Techniques developed to reduce baseline imbalance - for example, restricted randomisation using allocation by blocks with or without stratification – may deliver well-matched groups but only at the cost of jeopardizing the randomisation process.[11-13] The use of blocks provides an opportunity for researchers to predict future allocation based on knowledge of the treatment received by previously recruited patients and, although this is more likely in open studies, the potential for this is also present in double-blind trials. Hence, studies which reject simple randomisation in preference for more complex processes designed to reduce baseline imbalance should be viewed with caution.

Introduction of new relevant variables during a study

Even if randomisation is successful in the formation of well-matched groups, the equal distribution of relevant variables may be disrupted during the course of the study. Investigators who know which treatment each patient is receiving may behave differently depending on the treatment given.[21] Knowledge of treatment allocation raises the possibility of different groups being managed differently. There may, for example, be differences in the prescription of additional drugs, in the frequencies of investigations, in the response to clinical events and in decisions related to withdrawal of a patient from the study.

While the primary purpose of double-blind administration of medication is to eliminate bias in the assessment of the outcome on the part of patients and investigators, the technique also preserves randomisation by preventing the unequal distribution of relevant variables introduced during the study. However, blinding may simply be impossible: this is most obviously the case with surgical procedures but also applies to many other types of treatment including, for instance, orthopaedic traction, physiotherapy and psychotherapy. And, even when it is suitable, the double-blind technique may fail to conceal the treatment from patients or investigators. Physiological effects of drugs may inform the investigators of the treatment, for example, bradycardia with beta-blockers or tremor with salbutamol. If a drug has well-recognised and obvious adverse reactions - for example, the extra-pyramidal side-effects of phenothiazines or the facial changes associated with prednisolone - then the occurrence of these problems discloses the presence of the drug. There are also incidental features of certain drugs that signal their use - the orange colour of the urine of patients receiving rifampicin and the black discolouration of the stools in those taking iron or bismuth compounds being obvious examples. Finally, the double-blind process is susceptible to fraud: details of the actual treatment received by individual patients may be obtained by tampering with envelopes or breaking the randomisation codes, as well as testing tablets obtained while assessing compliance during follow-up visits.

It may be argued that while blinding is important in preventing bias related to soft end-points it may be dispensed with in studies with unambiguous, objective outcomes. However, the omission or failure of blinding weakens the assumption that groups formed by the randomisation process are equally matched for all relevant variables in the later stages of the study.

Disruption of randomisation during analysis

For a variety of reasons, members of the study population may be considered for exclusion from the final analysis. These include patients admitted to the study who are later identified as not meeting the entry criteria, those who develop the outcome before starting treatment, protocol violations – for example, patients failing to comply with treatment, receiving additional therapy or refusing subsequent investigations – those withdrawn because of adverse drug reactions or the development of other diseases, and those lost to follow-up. Exclusion of patients, however, should be avoided whenever possible.[22] Since it cannot be concluded that the reason for the exclusion is unrelated to relevant variables and, by implication, to the outcome of the study, the only way of preserving the randomisation process is to include all patients in an intention-to-treat analysis. This, however, is not possible in respect of patients lost to follow-up and their exclusion threatens the integrity of randomisation to a variable extent depending on the proportion of patients involved. Detailed information in publications regarding the intention-to-treat analysis and patients excluded, while frequently omitted,[22] is essential for accurate interpretation of the study.

Problems with Randomisation

Initial phase
- **Non-random mechanism**
- **Failure to conceal allocation**
- **Baseline imbalance**

Introduction of new relevant variables during study
- **Unequal management of different groups**
- **Failure of double-blind technique**

Disruption of randomisation during analysis
- **Failure to include all patient in the analysis**

In principle, randomisation offers a way of performing experiments in those conditions where there is inadequate knowledge of all the relevant variables contributing to the outcome. In practice, however, the process is often flawed.

Internal Validity of Clinical Trials

The internal validity of a clinical trial refers to the justification for the inference that the difference in outcome is due to the difference in treatment. This inference is valid only if alternative explanations - namely, the unequal distribution of other relevant variables among the treatment groups, the presence of bias in the assessment of the outcome and the difference being due to chance - have been excluded by the design, performance and analysis of the trial.[23]

Equal distribution of relevant variables

A valid randomisation process with attention to allocation concealment delivers groups that are well-matched in terms of relevant variables at the start of the study. Double-blind administration of treatment protects the randomisation process during the study period by preventing the introduction of relevant variables which are not equally distributed between the groups. And an intention-to-treat analysis reduces any disruption to randomisation process during the phase of data analysis. Provided these conditions are satisfied, it may be argued that any difference in outcome cannot be the result of differences in relevant variables among the groups other than the treatment under investigation.

Avoidance of bias in assessment of outcome

By ensuring that those involved in the study are unaware of the treatment received, bias in relation to the assessment of the outcome of a clinical trial – on the part of either the investigator or patient – may be avoided. Thus, not only is the double-blind technique important for preventing the unequal distribution of relevant variables during the trial but it is the primary means of protecting against bias. The type of outcome being assessed is of importance in considering the possibility of bias: hard end-points – such as mortality – are much less open to bias than soft end-points which may allow an element of interpretation.

Exclusion of chance

The role of statistics in medical research is to advise on the probability that the difference detected in the trial is due simply to chance. During recent decades, though, statistics have acquired an exaggerated importance. The clinical relevance of the results now takes second place to the assertion of statistical significance, while imperceptible differences between drug and placebo are obscured by boasts of low P-values. Researchers, editors of journals and the medical profession in general have become mesmerised by statistics while forgetting that statistical analysis is a minor player in medical research. The role of statistics is merely permissive, to nod affirmatively when the arithmetic indicates that chance is unlikely to explain the difference, thus allowing the more important business of judging the rest of the evidence, including the clinical relevance of the findings, to proceed.

Internal Validity

A difference in outcome may be attributed to a difference in treatment if the following have been excluded:

- **The effect of other known or unknown relevant variables**
- **Bias in the assessment of the outcome**
- **The results are due to chance**

Placebo Controls

In many ways, the placebo control is the most crucial component of clinical trials, although it must be said that nowadays its use is often abandoned in favour of comparative studies. Trials which involve a placebo control fulfil the requirements of classical variative induction. In other words, they potentially allow all the other circumstances to be held constant apart from the intervention under investigation. Thus, in clinical studies, the placebo control provides information concerning the outcome of patients in the absence of the active drug which is essential in a field where so much uncertainty exists.[24] Moreover, in non-comparative studies, the placebo control permits the use of double-blind administration of medication which avoids problems associated with bias.

In recent times, many studies comparing the effect of different therapies have dispensed with placebo controls. These studies usually involve a comparison between a new drug and a previously established treatment, and rely on a number of dubious assumptions. Firstly, it is assumed that the established therapy has a proven effect; however, in many cases the evidence in favour of this is either absent or is derived from inadequate studies performed at an earlier time. Secondly, it is assumed that the designers of the study select the most effective established therapy with which to compare the new drug; this, though, is often not the case. Finally, it is assumed that patients and their disease in the trial will behave in the same way as those in previous studies; again, there are no firm grounds to believe that this is the case. If a non-placebo comparative trial produces results which show that the new drug is as effective as established treatment, it is also likely to conclude that - given the above assumptions - the new drug would improve the outcome of untreated patients; this is clearly an unsubstantiated claim.

Placebo Controls

Crucial to clinical trials
- **Fulfil requirement of classical variative induction**
- **Provide data of the outcome in untreated patients**

Problems
- **Ethical constraints to the use of placebo**
- **Unwillingness of patients to participate**

Clinical trials without placebo controls are open to abuse. Consider the case of a promising new drug, developed at a cost of hundreds of millions of pounds, which is believed to have some advantages over established therapies in terms of side-effects and drug interactions. A comparator treatment is deliberately chosen because it is not the most effective of currently available treatments and has well recognised and frequent adverse drug reactions; the entry criteria for the study are selected so that patients with features suggestive of a poor response to therapy are excluded; and the threshold for a successful outcome to the study is lowered. Such manipulation of the study design is almost guaranteed to produce results that are favourable to the pharmaceutical company. But that is not all: the choice of a comparator drug with known, frequent side-effects threatens the integrity of the entire study. Double-blind administration is hampered by side-effects disclosing the presence of the comparator drug; this disrupts the preservation of randomisation and introduces the possibility of bias in the assessment of the outcome. In addition, the high frequency of side-effects in the comparator group encourages withdrawals, thus leading to disruption of randomisation during the stage of analysis.

Even if it were the case that clinical trials were designed and executed by those who were entirely impartial, the problems associated with comparative studies would still be present. However, given that most trials are conducted by those with a vested interest in the outcome, the avoidance of placebo controls severely compromises the results of such studies. The justification frequently cited for comparative trials is that the use of a placebo control is unethical in situations where an effective treatment is already available. While there are circumstances in which the use of placebo would be difficult to support, in many other circumstances placebo-controls would be reasonable. Moreover, as has recently been pointed out, it is legitimate to ask whether it is ethical to perform studies likely to yield unreliable results.[24]

External Validity of Clinical Trials

External validity concerns the justification for the assertion that the results of a clinical trial are applicable to a wider population than simply those patients participating in the study.[23] At this point, it is worth noting that if the internal validity is poor, then there is little point in considering the external validity. However, once the internal validity has been established, an assessment of external validity should follow.

Consider an assessment of the external validity of the conclusion to a study stating that "drug X reduces the mortality of patients with disease Y". The conclusion is valid only if the study population is representative of the whole population of patients with disease Y. However, unless the selection of patients is completely random, there will inevitably be differences between the group of patients recruited to the trial and the general population of patients with disease Y. The external validity of the conclusion, therefore, will depend on the extent - and relevance - of these differences. For example, the results of a study that included only patients with a mild form of disease Y clearly could not legitimately be applied to patients with moderate or severe disease.

The ways in which the study population differ from the general population of patients with disease Y depends on the methods of selection, usually referred to as the inclusion and exclusion criteria. These criteria refer to characteristics both of the patients and the disease. In some cases, these characteristics will be recognised as being relevant to the outcome, whereas in other cases their relevance will be unknown. However, regardless of whether the relevance of these characteristics is known or unknown, questions immediately arise concerning the external validity.

Strictly speaking, the results of a study may only be applied to similar patients with similar disease given similar treatment in a similar setting. Thus the conclusion "drug X reduces the mortality in disease Y" is misleading. It should be regarded as a shorthand version, made available merely as a temporary expedient, of a much more detailed statement which includes complete definitions of all the terms and which is to be used whenever the conclusion is to be applied in practice. For example, a more accurate specification of the conclusion might read: "drug X (.... doses, route of administration, frequency, timing, relation to meals, duration....) reduces the mortality in patients (age range...., without other specified co-existent diseases...., not receiving other specified medication...., with no known allergy to certain specified compounds, excluding females of child-bearing age, who agreed to participate in the study and were able to give informed consent....) with disease Y (diagnosed by specified criteria...., including those only of mild or moderate severity, excluding those with specified complications....) in the setting of a clinical trial (involving a specified protocol for observations, other interventions etc). That the practical consequences of an accurate specification of the conclusion are inconvenient is no justification for the use of misleading generalisations.

External Validity

Depends on:

- **Selection of study population (inclusion/exclusion criteria)**

- **Effect of participation in study**

- **Wording of the study conclusion**

The importance of the effect of the setting within a trial is often overlooked.[25] Clinical trials are usually performed by doctors with a particular interest in the disease and in units with considerable expertise, including nurses with specialist skills and well-qualified junior staff; under such circumstances, the standard of care would be expected to be high. The investigators often have a financial incentive - either personally or in respect of their unit - to manage the study diligently. For instance, payments from the pharmaceutical companies of more than one thousand pounds per patient recruited are not unusual.[26] Furthermore, as the investigators know that their actions will be scrutinised when the record books are examined, there will be a tendency to ensure that medication is given according to the specifications in the protocol, that symptoms are promptly treated and that complications are identified early and managed swiftly. The nurses, too, will be aware of the study requirements for regular observations which may result in detection of complications earlier than in the normal course of events. Thus, there are reasons to believe that patients may receive a different standard of care in the course of a clinical trial than would otherwise have been the case in routine clinical practice.

The purpose of clinical trials is to identify generalisations that are applicable to large groups of patients with particular diseases. Trials involve individual patients and these individuals have many different characteristics. One of the principles of the scientific method is that any reference class - that is, the group or collection of items about which a general statement is to be made - should be restricted to the most homogeneous class available. Thus, according to this principle, inclusion and exclusion criteria for recruitment into the study should be chosen so as to produce as homogeneous a class as possible. However, the rigorous application of such criteria excludes a large proportion of patients with the disease. As a result, it would not be legitimate to apply any generalisation derived from a homogeneous study population to the whole population of patients with the disease. Thus, there is a paradox: the closer the design of a clinical trial complies with the scientific principle of homogeneous reference classes, the more the external validity of the trial will be threatened if the conclusions are to be applied to the general population of patients with the disease in question.

Evidence of Flaws in Published Randomised Trials

In principle, a well-designed and correctly executed double-blind, randomised controlled trial should have a high degree of internal validity such that differences in outcome may be attributed to treatment effects. In practice, such confidence in the results of randomised clinical trials is misplaced.

Criticism of clinical trials has centred on the failure of studies to adhere to the basic principles of randomised controlled trials. The findings of literature reviews investigating the standard of randomised controlled trials in a number of branches of medicine have been disappointing.[27-31] For example, an extensive review of the literature involving 2000 clinical trials relating to the treatment of schizophrenia gives cause for concern.[31] The results reflected poorly on the standard of clinical research: two-thirds of trials were of low quality and there was no evidence of improvement over time. In general, poor quality studies were associated with an increased estimate of the therapeutic benefit. The use of haloperidol as a control was common, despite the fact that its well-recognised and frequent side-effects would impair blinding and lead to bias, as well as showing the newer drug in a more favourable light. The conclusion by the authors that '...*the findings of this survey are as bad, if not worse, as those of other disciplines of health care"* would appear to be entirely justified.

It is well known that details of the method of randomisation,[11] of allocation concealment,[13] of blinding techniques[21] and of the handling of exclusions[22] are frequently absent from published trials. A recent study, for example, reported that allocation concealment was adequate in only 25%, that blinding was unsatisfactory in 20% and that an intention-to-treat analysis was used in only 55% of randomised controlled trials.[32]

In the 1980's, Rennie wrote scathingly about the standard of studies published in medical journals: *"There seems to be no study too fragmented, no hypothesis too trivial, no literature citation too biased or too egotistical, no design too warped, no methodology too bungled, no presentation of results too inaccurate, too obscure and too contradictory, no analysis too self-serving, no argument too circular, no conclusions too trifling or too unjustified, and no grammar and syntax too offensive for a paper to end up in print."* [33] In the 1990's, Altman commented on *"the scandal of poor medical research"* [34] A decade later, concern continues to be expressed about the quality of published clinical trials[35,36]

These problems may be traced to various parts of the research process.[37] As much of medical research is performed by clinicians who have little training in the necessary skills, including design and analysis of trials, it is hardly surprising that errors are commonplace. Research ethics committees have a responsibility to assess the scientific merit of proposed studies and to reject those which fail to meet the required standards yet the poor quality of many studies suggests that they are not fulfilling this role. The editors of journals, too, have a duty to ensure that papers submitted for publication are carefully reviewed by those with the appropriate expertise. In this regard, the evidence indicates that statistical review occurs in only a minority of cases.

Conclusions

Given the differences among both patients and their diseases, together with the recognition that the relevance of such differences to the outcome of clinical trials is mostly unknown, it is only to be expected that medical researchers find the allure of randomisation irresistible. By adopting this process, the clinical trial appears - at a stroke - to be free of the criticism that any difference in outcome might be due to factors other than the difference in treatment. In addition, the introduction of double-blind administration further enhances the internal validity of clinical trials by preserving the randomisation process and preventing bias in the assessment of the outcome.

In theory, at least, the randomised controlled trial appears to offer a solution to the problem of heterogeneity. However, the methodology is complex and, at every stage, errors may occur including faults with the initial random allocation of treatment, the failure to preserve the equal distribution of relevant variables throughout the study period and the disruption of the randomisation process during data analysis. The evidence from studies investigating the quality of published randomised trials suggests that the conditions for internal validity are seldom satisfied in full.

As every randomised trial selects patients according to predetermined inclusion and exclusion criteria, differences between those recruited to the study and the wider population of patients are inevitable. Moreover, the special circumstances surrounding clinical trials cannot be discounted when projecting the results of a study to a wider population of patients. Thus, the external validity of randomised trials is always open to challenge.

Both internal and external validity are, therefore, compromised in randomised clinical trials. The proposed solutions to the problems of internal validity focus on encouraging compliance with a set of rules such as those described by the CONSORT group,[35] ensuring that research is carried out only by those trained for that purpose and strengthening the checks and balances by persuading research ethics committees, the editors of journal and referees to meet their responsibilities by scrutinizing clinical trials with the utmost care.[37]

Underlying this approach, there seems to be the assumption that the problems of randomised controlled trials are grounded in human error alone, that they may be eradicated by a concerted campaign of education and that, provided researchers as well as those involved in checking their work behave correctly, all will be well and clinical research will yield reliable generalisations. But this is a one-sided analysis. It is a case of blaming the workman without any regard to the quality of his tools. An alternative interpretation is that the sheer complexity of randomised trials impedes compliance with all of the conditions required for internal validity. Indeed, the methodology is so unwieldy that it seems unlikely that full compliance would ever be achieved on a regular basis. And the reliability of the results is so dependent upon compliance at every stage of the process that a single error or omission may bring the whole enterprise into question.

If the practice of randomised trials so frequently fails to meet the requirements for the demonstration of internal and external validity, then perhaps the fault lies in the methodology itself. But such a conclusion is seemingly anathema to those involved in medical research who view the randomised controlled trial as sacrosanct. Indeed, the randomised trial is so entrenched in the minds of researchers that is has become, to use Kuhn's terminology, a paradigm and, as such, must not be the subject of doubt. Nonetheless, doubts about the methodology cannot be ignored, especially when the focus turns to large-scale randomised trials.

References

1. Mill JS. *A System of Logic*. Longmans, Green & Co. London, 1884. Bk III; Chap VII; Sect 1; P248.

2. Mill JS. *A System of Logic*. Longmans, Green & Co. London, 1884. Bk III; Chap VIII.

3. Fibiger J. Om Serumbehandling af Difteri. *Hospitalstidende* 1898;6;309-25,337-50.

4. Hrobjartsson A, Gotsche PC, Gluud C. The controlled clinical trial turns 100 years: Fibiger's trial of serum treatment of diphtheria. *Br Med J* 1998;317;1243-5.

5. Amberson JB, McMahon BL, Pinner MA. A clinical trial of sanocrysin in pulmonary tuberculosis. *Amer Rev Tuberc* 1931;24;401-35.

6. Medical Research Council Therapeutic Trials Committee. The serum treatment of lobar pneumonia. *BrMed J* 1934;i;241-5.

7. Medical Research Council Patulin Trials Committee. Clinical trial of patulin in the common cold. *Lancet* 1944;ii;373-4.

8. Medical Research Council Whooping-Cough Immunization Committee. The prevention of whooping-cough by vaccination. *Br Med J* 1951;i;1463-71.

9. MRC Streptomycin in Tuberculosis Trials Committee. Streptomycin treatment for pulmonary tuberculosis. *Br Med J* 1948;ii;769-82.

10. Hill AB. Principles of medical statistics: I. The aim of the statistical method. *Lancet* 1937;I;41-3.

11. Schulz KF & Grimes DA. Generation of allocation sequences in randomised trials: chance, no choice. *Lancet* 2002;259;515-19.

12. Torgerson DJ, Roberts C. Randomisation methods: concealment. *Br J Med* 1999;319;375-6.

13. Schulz KF & Grimes DA. Allocation concealment in randomised trials: defending against deciphering. *Lancet* 2002;359;614-18.

14. Schulz KF & Grimes DA. Unequal group sizes in randomised trials: guarding against guessing. *Lancet* 2002;359;966-70.

15. Roberts C & Torgerson DJ. Baseline imbalance in randomised controlled trials. *Br Med J* 1999;319;185.

16. Roberts C, Torgerson D. Randomisation methods in controlled trials. *Br Med J* 1998;317;1301.

17. Sleight P et al. for the Heart Outcomes Prevention Evaluation (HOPE) Study Investigators. Blood pressure reduction and cardiovascular risk in HOPE study. *Lancet* 2001;358;2130-1.

18. Lindholm LH et al. Cardiovascular morbidity and mortality in patients with diabetes in the Losartan Intervention for Endpoint reduction in hypertension study (LIFE): randomised trial against atenolol. *Lancet* 2002;359;1004-10.

19. Taylor R. Blood pressure and cardiovascular risk in the HOPE study. *Lancet* 2002;359;2117-8.

20. Bloom JM. Losartan for cardiovascular disease in patients with and without diabetes in the LIFE study. *Lancet* 2002;359;2201.

21. Schulz KF & Grimes DA. Blinding in randomised trials: hiding who got what. *Lancet* 2002;359;696-700.

22. Schulz KF & Grimes DA. Sample size slippages in randomised trials: exclusions and the lost and wayward. *Lancet* 2002;359;781-85.

23. Elwood JM. *Causal Relationships in Medicine.* Oxford Medical Publications, 1988.

24. Tramer MR, Reynolds DJM, Moore RA, McQuay HJ. When placebo controlled trials are essential and equivalence trials are inadequate. *Br Med J* 1998;317;875-80.

25. Braunholtz DA, Edwards SJ, Lilford RJ. Are randomised clinical trials good for us (in the short term)? Evidence for a "trial effect". *J Clin Epidemiol* 2001;54;217-24.

26. Rao JN & Cassia LJS. Ethics of undisclosed payments to doctors recruiting patients in clinical trials. *Br Med J* 2002;325;36-7.

27. Nicolucci A, Grilli R, Alexanian AA, et al. Quality, evolution, and clinical implications of randomised, controlled trials on the treatment of lung cancer. A lost opportunity for meta-analysis. *JAMA* 1989;262;2101-7.

28. Vandekerckhove P, O'Donovan PA, Lilford RJ, et al. Infertility treatment: from cookery to science. The epidemiology of randomised controlled trials. *Br J Obstet Gynaecol* 1993;100;1005-36.

29. Cheng K, Smyth RL, Motley J, et al. Randomised controlled trials in cystic fibrosis (1966-1997) categorised by time, design, and intervention.. *Pediatr Pulmonol* 2000;29;1-7.

30. Moher D, Pharm B, Jones A, et al. Does quality of reports of randomised trials affect estimates of intervention efficacy reported in meta-analyses? *Lancet* 1998;352;609-13.

31. Thornley B & Adams C. Content and quality of 2000 controlled trials in schizophrenia over 50 years. *Br Med J* 1998;317;1181-4.

32. Huwiler-Muntener K, Juni P, Junker C, Egger M. Quality of reporting of randomised trials as a measure of methodologic quality. *JAMA* 2002;287;2801-4.

33. Rennie D. Guarding the guardians. *JAMA* 1986;256;2391-2

34. Altman DG. The scandal of poor medical research. *Br Med J* 1994;308;283-4.

35. Moher D, Schulz KF, Altman DG. The CONSORT statement: revised recommendations for improving the quality of reports of parallel-group randomised trials. *Lancet* 2001;357;1191-94.

36. Altman DG, Schulz KF, Moher D, et al. The revised CONSORT statement for reporting randomised trials: explanation and elaboration. *Ann Intern Med* 2001;134;663-94.

37. Altman DG. Poor quality medical research: what can journals do? *JAMA* 2002;287;2765-7.

IV

LARGE-SCALE RANDOMISED TRIALS – FULL OF SOUND AND FURY, SIGNIFYING NOTHING?

In principle, the methodology of large-scale randomised trials is no different from that of smaller studies. Consequently, the potential flaws described in the previous chapter are shared equally among randomised trials regardless of the number of patients participating. This is not to say that their effects are of similar importance; on the contrary, minor problems relating to the randomisation process, for instance, have greater impact in mega-trials than in smaller studies. Similarly, problems associated with external validity are of greater concern in larger trials. In general, the weaknesses of smaller randomised controlled trials become more serious in context of mega-trials.

There are, though, certain features peculiar to mega-trials that create further problems. The purpose of these studies is the recruitment of a large number of patients in order to bestow statistical significance upon a small treatment difference. Thus, every mega-trial reports only a small difference between the treatment groups and this has important implications. For example, it raises questions about the validity of causal inference and about the meaning of the results to individual patients.

A further aspect of mega-trials is the way in which the methodology is far removed from that of science. Indeed, such are the differences between the two that it is reasonable to view mega-trials as a distinct approach to the investigation of phenomena in the natural world. And, this, of course, implies that mega-trials must justify their validity independently. As will be shown, this is a far from easy task.

From Science to Large-Scale Clinical Trials

In terms of the reliability of generalisations – and, hence, their practical applications – there is a spectrum of results ranging from those produced by the experiments of the physical sciences, through those of the life sciences including the more basic parts of medical research, to those of large-scale randomised trials.

Consider the case of a new chemical compound and its relationship to the freezing point of water. Perhaps this compound was accidentally added to the water in containers left outside in the winter and that it was subsequently observed that the water failed to freeze. Alternatively, the similarities in chemical structure between the new compound and ethylene glycol may have raised the question about its use as an anti-freeze, encouraged by the lower cost of production or the absence of toxicity of the new compound. Whether the hypothesis that the compound lowers the freezing point of water is derived from observation instances or from pre-existing theory, a formal controlled experiment is designed to test its validity. Two identical beakers containing x millilitres of pure water are placed in a refrigerator at $0^{o}C$ for y hours. To one of the beakers has been added z grams of the compound. Precise definitions of all the materials, the equipment, the standardisation procedures and the methods ensure that the initial conditions are exactly the same for each beaker apart from the addition of the compound. Repeated experiments show that on every occasion the water freezes only in the beaker without the compound. Under such circumstances, the hypothesis is confirmed. Subsequent experiments, for example, the construction of dose-response curves at varying concentrations and temperatures, again subject the hypothesis to testing and the results provide further support for the hypothesis. Moreover, the background theory to these experiments includes the known effects of other chemical compounds on the freezing point of water. Given all of this evidence, we may infer from repeated observations of the failure of water containing the compound to freeze at $0^{\circ}C$ to the generalisation that the compound reduces the freezing point of water.

But, what if someone were to insist that the only way to prove the hypothesis is to perform a randomised controlled trial, perhaps justifying himself by speculating that other factors may be responsible for the observed phenomenon? Such an experiment would be easy to design and execute but would it really add anything the to results of the original studies? Given the homogeneity of the results, there is no requirement for randomisation – that is, there are no known or unknown relevant variables that are unequally distributed and require to be distributed equally.

Now, imagine the same individual protesting that there is no proof that vitamin B_{12} successfully treats pernicious anaemia: is his demand for a randomised trial justifiable? Would there be anything to be gained by performing such a study in patients with macrocytic anaemia, megaloblastic bone marrow, low serum B_{12} levels, gastric parietal cell and intrinsic factor antibodies, and achlorhydria? This treatment has, after all, been used in numerous patients over many decades and the vast majority respond with a reticulocytosis followed by a rise in haemoglobin to within the normal range while it is well established that such patients do not experience a spontaneous resolution. Surely, as in the case of compound C and the freezing point of water, there is no requirement for randomisation in the presence of homogeneity?

But what about situations in which heterogeneity is a feature of both treated and untreated groups of patients? Consider a clinical trial of a new proton pump inhibitor in patients with duodenal ulcers. Without randomisation, 200 patients are divided into two groups, one of which receives the drug and the other is left without treatment. After a specified period of time, duodenal ulcers are found to have healed in 95% of patients receiving the drug compared with only 35% of the control group. Surely these results support the conclusion that the new drug is beneficial to patients with duodenal ulcers? Moreover, this conclusion is supported by extensive background knowledge. For example, numerous studies have shown that approximately one-third of duodenal ulcers heal spontaneously, that duodenal ulcers are related to acid secretion – they are associated with hypersecretion of hydrochloric acid and do not occur in patients with achlorhydria – that proton pump inhibitors greatly reduce acid secretion, that members of this class of drugs currently in use heal more than 90% of duodenal ulcers and that the rates of healing with all types of gastric anti-secretory drugs are proportional to the degree of acid suppression. Thus, the results of the trial may be readily accommodated within our pre-existing knowledge of duodenal ulcer disease and the mechanisms of healing.

In these circumstances, is randomisation necessary? Of course, it is possible that the two groups were not matched at the start of the study and that the untreated group comprised a much higher proportion of patients with factors likely to inhibit ulcer healing but, unless there was a deliberate policy to allocate certain types of patients to one particular group, this explanation is implausible given the large treatment difference. It should also be remembered that randomisation is no guarantee that research misconduct will not occur. Randomisation may offer peace of mind to some, but it makes little material difference to the value of the study. Any doubts would, in any case, be dispelled by subsequent clinical experience: if the results of the trial are valid, then the drug will make a substantial difference as the ulcers will persist in most untreated patients while they will be healed in nearly all patients receiving the medication.

Arguments in favour of randomisation increase in potency as the size of the absolute difference diminishes. Nowhere is this more obvious than in the case of large-scale randomised controlled trials. These studies, often involving tens of thousands of patients, relate to the common chronic diseases – for example, ischaemic heart disease - which are the leading causes of illness and death. Large numbers of patients have to be recruited to these trials because the outcomes occur in only a small proportion of patients and the drugs under investigation have only a limited effect in preventing the outcomes. The consequence of these two features is that the studies produce, at best, only a small difference between the treatment groups and, if this is to be shown to be statistically significant, thousands of patients must be included. Without randomisation, there would be no possibility of arguing that the small difference was not the result of minor differences in the distribution of relevant variables between the groups.

Mega-trials have an enormous influence on the long-term management of millions of patients. They are the impetus to the expenditure of billions of pounds and, as a result, place a huge burden on scarce resources of health care systems. Furthermore, for the pharmaceutical companies, they are the source of vast fortunes. Against this background, it is of the utmost importance that the methodology of mega-trials is sound and that the results are valid. This, though, is far from being the case.

Causal Inference in Mega-trials

If we set to one side the potential problems with randomisation that threaten the internal validity, more subtle challenges remain to causal inference in large-scale randomised trials. These have their origin in the heterogeneity of the study population and the absence of regularity, both of which bring any causal inference into question.

The regularity theory

Consider the case of a hypothetical mega-trial designed to determine the effect of a new drug Y on the mortality from disease X. After the application of inclusion and exclusion criteria, 20,000 patients with disease X were randomised to receive either drug Y or placebo continuously for a period of five years. Let us assume that the randomisation process contained no flaws, that the double-blind technique successfully prevented any disclosure of medication, that the analysis included all patients randomised at the start of the study and that the difference was statistically significant – in other words, that the conditions for internal validity were satisfied. The results showed that the mortality in patients receiving drug Y was 6%, compared with 7% in those receiving placebo. The conclusion was reached that drug Y reduced mortality by 14% in patients with disease X.

In these circumstances, is the conclusion of the study valid? Do the data support the claim for a causal link between drug Y and the reduction in mortality from disease X? On the basis of the regularity theory, it is difficult to justify this inference. To begin with, there are two phenomena involved in this study. The first concerns the mortality of untreated patients with disease X; the second, relates to the effect of drug Y on those patients with disease X who would have died if left untreated. This is a simplified analysis because further phenomena may be involved, such as patients who died as a result of taking drug Y rather than the disease itself, but for the purpose of this discussion they may ignored. The first phenomenon – observed in the placebo group and constituting the "background conditions" – clearly demonstrates the presence of heterogeneity for relevant variables with respect to the outcome since only *some* untreated patients died. The placebo group, therefore, comprises a minimum of two subgroups, the 7% who died (subgroup (a)) and the 93% who survived (subgroup (b)). Given that the relevant variables are equally distributed by randomisation, the group receiving drug Y is also made up of subgroups (a) and (b). However, within subgroup (a), there is also heterogeneity in respect of the outcome in the presence of drug Y because it comprises the 6% who died (subgroup (c)) and the 1% who survived (subgroup (d)). Thus, each phenomenon displays both heterogeneity and an absence of regularity.

As discussed earlier, a regular association between one event and another depends on the presence of a homogeneous reference class. The use of randomisation entails that the study population is heterogeneous in respect of relevant variables. In the physical sciences, for example, there is no prospect of unequal distribution of relevant variables because all objects and events are the same in terms of the outcome and the only relevant variable unequally distributed is the factor under investigation. But, although randomisation distributes the relevant variables equally, it does not remove the heterogeneity nor does it deliver regularity. How, then, is causation established?

If causal inference regarding the effect of drug Y on mortality is to be based on the regularity theory, then it must refer to regularity residing in subgroup (d), that is, in those patients who would have died but survived due to treatment. Subgroup (d), of course, is derived from subgroups (a) and (c), each of which are defined only by the outcome. Hence, any generalisation about the effect of drug Y on subgroup (d) is derived from causal inference concerning a reference class which cannot be identified in advance of the outcome. Such an approach is contrary to the usual understanding of causation - a causal generalisation is derived from observation instances in which the reference class is identified independently of the outcome.

Thus, causal inference based on data relating to the entire study population is flawed because of the absence of any regularity. On the other hand, if attention turns to the underlying subgroups, then causal inference is flawed because of a failure to identify the reference class. Mega-trials, therefore, cannot use the regularity theory as the basis for causal inference. But this theory is the foundation for our concepts of causation, in everyday life as well as in science. What, then, is the basis for causal inference in mega-trials?

Causal inference – an alternative approach
The 19th century was a time of dramatic discoveries in medicine, especially in the field of microbiology with the identification of many of the pathogenic bacteria. In an attempt to establish a causal relationship between a particular organism and a specific disease, Jacob Henle described a set of postulates which were later modified by his pupil, Robert Koch.[1] Comprising a set of universal statements which entailed, amongst other things, that the

putative cause should be present in all instances of the disease, the Henle-Koch postulates were too rigid and too impractical to survive for long. By the mid-twentieth century, they were replaced by what have become known as the epidemiological criteria for causation. The landmark publication by the US Surgeon General in 1964 relating to smoking and health described the criteria by which causation was to be established.[2]

Most accounts of the epidemiological criteria for causation include the strength of the association, the specificity, temporal priority, consistency across different studies, coherence with pre-existing facts and theory, evidence from "natural" or unintentional experiments and the presence of a biological gradient between the putative cause and its effect.[2-5] Some criteria are recognised to have greater importance than others. Epidemiological data that show a strong association, consistency and a dose-response effect are considered to be convincing evidence of a causal relationship. This was the case, for example in the demonstration by Doll and Hill of the link between smoking and lung cancer.[6] Natural experiments, too, strongly support causation, as in the observations by John Snow of the cholera epidemics in London in the mid-nineteenth century.[7] On the other side, the absence of either temporal priority or consistency and, to a lesser extent, a lack of coherence argue against any causal relationship.

But, while the epidemiological criteria may suggest causation, indicate the direction of future research and even provide the basis for action, they are never sufficient to prove a causal relationship. Austin Bradford Hill summarised this position succinctly: *"None of [the criteria] can bring indisputable evidence for or against the cause and effect hypothesis and none can be required as a sine qua non... What they can do, with greater or less strength, is to help us make up our minds..."* [3]

However, while all of the criteria are relevant to causal inference, the strength of the association - measured by the relative risk or odds ratio - has assumed pre-eminence. The epidemiological approach centres on the establishment of a statistical relationship between the supposed cause and its effect. As Susser stated: *"In epidemiology, we recognise the possible presence of a cause by its coincidence, beyond the bounds of chance, with the effect or change...the suspect factor and the outcome are statistically associated."* [8]   In other words, causation – in the context of epidemiological studies – is nothing but the demonstration of a statistically significant association.

But the notion of statistical causation has been taken up by clinical research and used in the interpretation of randomised controlled trials. Indeed, there are similarities between epidemiological studies and mega-trials: both usually involve large numbers of individuals, both compare outcomes which occur at a low frequency in two or more groups, and both ultimately judge the presence of a causal relationship in terms of a small – but statistically significant - difference in outcome between the groups. There are, of course, notable differences: randomisation and the direct manipulation of the relevant variable under investigation in clinical trials leads to greater internal validity than is present in the observational studies. However, the foundation of each type of study is an acceptance of causation in terms of a statistically significant difference.

In both epidemiological studies and mega-trials, the underlying causal reasoning is the same: the first step is the elimination of confounding and bias – in one case using carefully selected controls, in the other using randomisation and blinding; the second step is the demonstration of a statistical association between exposure and outcome; finally, the inference is made that the relationship is one of causation. Such an argument, based on the exclusion of alternative explanations, is contrary to the scientific approach to causation which is defined in positive terms by observing a regular association between objects or events. In the absence of regularity between the drug and the outcome, all that is left for mega-trials – like epidemiological studies – is to seek out marginal differences between the groups against a background of heterogeneity.

It is clear that the concept of causation derived from the statistical approach differs in meaning from that in everyday life or science. In terms of the methods and criteria by which they are defined, the two concepts of causation are patently distinct. More important, however, are the differences in use and practical applications of the concepts. A causal generalisation of science applies to any individual instance; hence, it allows accurate prediction. In contrast, the conclusion of a mega-trial fails to support any prediction concerning the effect of treatment on an individual patient. For example, statements such as "if the treatment were to be given, the patient would survive" or "if the patient had not been given the treatment, then he would not have survived" are not supported by the data from mega-trials. On the other hand, these subjunctives and counterfactual conditionals are fully licensed by the generalisations of science and may be used to explain what we normally understand by the concept of causation.

The way we view a causal generalisation – that is, the confidence we have in its reliability – differs when we consider the two concepts. A scientific statement, based on the results of unequivocal observations under experimental conditions, is readily accepted. To doubt it would be to bring into question the very means by which we obtain knowledge of causal relationships in the natural world. The situation, though, is very different when it comes to causation based on the statistical approach. In this case, we may, for instance, ask why we should accept that a small difference in outcome tentatively linked by sophisticated statistical techniques to treatment is sufficient to establish the presence of a causal relationship. In fact, we have few qualms about dismissing the results of randomised trials when the results are unpalatable. Consider, for example, the extraordinary paper published in the *British Medical Journal* which reported the effects of prayer on patients with bacteraemia.[9] All patients with positive blood cultures at a university hospital in Israel between 1990 and 1996 were identified; in 2000 (four years after the last patient had been admitted), all 3393 patients were randomised into two groups, one receiving prayer for full recovery, the other having no active intervention. While mortality was similar in both groups, retroactive prayer produced statistically significant reductions in the duration of fever and length of hospital stay. The results should, of course, be dismissed on the grounds that the intervention occurred years after the outcome, thus defying the basic principle that a cause precedes its effect. Yet, the study was performed with due attention to the requirements for internal validity and the fact that its results may be disregarded shows that we do not feel obliged to accept the conclusions of this methodology in the same way that we do those produced by science.

Causation in mega-trials differs from that in science. We know what a causal generalisation entails in science, we understand how to use it and believe in its validity. In contrast, causal reasoning in mega-trials is obscure and unreliable.

External Validity of Mega-trials

As already discussed, the external validity of a clinical trial depends both on the study population closely resembling the wider population of patients with the disease in terms of those factors which affect the outcome and on the degree to which participation in the study by itself affects the outcome.

Given that patients recruited to randomised trials comprise a heterogeneous group, only a proportion of patients will develop the outcome. The size of this proportion, however, is important. For example, if 90% of controls develop the outcome and this proportion is reduced to 20% by the drug under investigation, then 70% of the patients have benefited from the treatment and, in such circumstances, it would be very unlikely that the treatment effect would be annulled by minor differences between those recruited to the study and the wider population. However, if only 8% of the controls developed the outcome compared with 6% of those receiving the drug, the external validity is brought into question by even small differences between the study group and the wider population. Thus, mega-trials face an almost inevitable challenge to their external validity directly as a consequence of the small treatment difference.

Patients excluded from mega-trials		
	Number of eligible patients	Patients excluded
ASSET study[10]	13,318	62%
GISSI-2 study[11]	38,086	67%
GISSI-3 study[12]	43,047	55%

Published mega-trials usually contain a long list of inclusion and exclusion criteria by which the study population is defined. This practice is clearly seen in the large studies of therapy in ischaemic heart disease and results in the exclusion of a substantial proportion of patients. For example, in both the ASSET study[10] and the GISSI-2 study[11], approximately two-thirds of patients were excluded before randomisation. While the reasons in the majority of these patients concerned the timing of their symptoms in relation to the treatment, a significant proportion was excluded on other grounds. In any case, regardless of the reason, the exclusion of patients threatens the external validity of the study. This conclusion is supported by the GISSI-3 study[12] in which only 45% of 43,047 patients admitted to coronary care units were randomised and the mortality in patients excluded from the study was more than twice that observed in those participating in the trial.

Of course, it would be possible to stipulate the precise population to which the results are applicable but this would depend on accurate specification of the inclusion and exclusion criteria. However, the frequent vagueness of some of the criteria, which inevitable allows interpretation, precludes any consistent definition of the study population.

Imprecise Exclusion Criteria	
ASSET study[10] LATE study[13]	"serious organic or psychiatric disease"
ISIS-2 study[14]	"absolute" or "possible" contraindications "some other life-threatening disease"
ISIS-3 study[15]	"not specified by the protocol but by the responsible physician"
ASSENT-2 study[16]	"any other disorder that the investigator judged would place the patient at increased risk"

The importance of criteria used to select patients for recruitment into studies cannot be exaggerated. A recent study from two district general hospitals which participated in mega-trials of thrombolysis reported that only 21% of patients with myocardial infarction were actually recruited to the trials[17]. The mortality in those patients participating in the mega-trials was 8%, compared with 18% in those excluded, suggesting that high risk patients were omitted from such studies and, hence, that any inference from the results to the general population of patients would be invalid.

The HOPE study[18], which investigated the effects of an angiotensin converting enzyme inhibitor in patients who were at high risk of cardiovascular disease, presented an even greater challenge to the external validity of mega-trials. After the application of inclusion and exclusion criteria, 10,576 eligible patients were identified. However, before randomisation, patients participated in a "run-in" phase of two weeks during which time they received the study drug, ramipril, followed by placebo. Ten percent of patients were subsequently excluded because of problems occurring during the run-in phase including non-compliance, side effects, increased creatinine and hyperkalaemia - all likely to be related more to the active drug than to placebo; the remaining 9541 patients entered the randomisation process. The results showed only minor benefits from treatment over the follow-up period of five years: the absolute difference in the primary outcome (a composite of myocardial infarction or stroke or death from cardiovascular disease) between ramipiril and placebo was only 3.8%, while the difference in the overall mortality was a mere 1.8%. Under these circumstances, the external validity of the study is severely eroded by the decision to incorporate the run-in phase as this process excluded patients for reasons that are of potential relevance to the clinical outcome.

External validity is a complex relationship between the study population and the wider population of patients with the disease in question. The smaller the absolute treatment difference, the greater is the potential threat to the external validity.

The Size of the Treatment Effect

Large-scale randomised controlled trials are designed precisely in those situations where a small treatment effect is expected. Indeed, the size of the study population is a direct indication of the size of the expected treatment difference. Thus, from studies involving many thousands of patients, it may be inferred that the effect of treatment is, at best, marginal. For instance, in the LIPID study[19], which involved more than 9000 patients observed for up to six years, the absolute reduction in mortality in patients receiving pravastatin was only 3.1%. Similarly, in the CARE study[20] – again involving pravastatin – the absolute reduction in the risk of stroke during five years of follow-up was only 1.2%. Other large-scale randomised trials in cardiovascular disease – such as those studying the effects of angiotensin converting enzyme inhibitors (for example, the GISSI-3 study[12] and the HOPE study[18]) or thrombolytic therapy (for example the ISIS-2 study[14]) – also report very small absolute differences.

It is, therefore, typical of mega-trials that they demonstrate only small treatment differences and this characteristic is the source of many of the flaws inherent in this methodology.

Small differences and causal inference

The criticism of causal inference in terms of the absence of regularity in mega-trials is augmented by the small treatment differences. The unequivocal causal relationships of science – where the outcome always occurs in the presence, but never in the absence, of the causal factor – are not applicable to mega-trials. Even accepting the inevitable presence of heterogeneity in the biological sciences, clinically relevant results such as the occurrence of the outcome in 70% of cases exposed to the causal factor compared with 10% of those unexposed, are no longer on offer. Instead, we are left to ponder a paltry difference in outcome of perhaps one or two percent between the active treatment and placebo. In such circumstances, our grasp of causal concepts seems to slip. As we pass along the spectrum from the physical sciences to mega-trials, our certainty about causal relationships fades until, faced with small differences in outcome, it disappears altogether.

Small differences in the context of flawed methodology

Against the background of uncertainty that accompanies mega-trials – including, for example, the many potential errors in the randomisation process - the size of the difference further undermines the value of the results. While a large absolute treatment difference of 70%, for instance, would support a claim for efficacy of a new drug even in a non-randomised study, a small difference of 3% is susceptible to challenge on the grounds that minor errors in the randomisation process might account for this finding. For instance, baseline imbalance arising purely from chance may contribute to the observed difference. Put simply, the smaller the difference, the more closely we are obliged to search for methodological errors; and, the smaller the difference, the less confident we may be in assuming that our search has excluded all errors.

Small differences in clinical practice

It is, perhaps, one the strangest aspects of mega-trials that the supposed benefits of a drug are not observable in routine clinical practice. Given that thousands of patients were required to show any difference, no single clinician would be able to treat a sufficient number of patients in order to detect the difference reported in the studies. Thus, as far as the clinician's experience is concerned, it makes no difference whether or not the result of a mega-trial is valid. This strange state of affairs is, of course, contrary to all notions of causation, whether in everyday life or in science.

Small differences and individual patients

The problems in communicating numerical information to patients are well recognised.[21] But, even if difficulties with the understanding of percentages or proportions are set aside, deeper problems about the appreciation of small treatment differences remain. For instance, what would it mean to an individual if he were told that the five-year mortality from his disease was 7%? The answer does not lie in some conversion of a percentage to a proportion, for a similar question may be asked of the new term. Surely the question concerns the importance which the patient attaches to a risk of 7%. And we will find this out by what he subsequently says and how he acts. He may, for example, look relieved and exclaim that he had thought he had little chance of being alive next year. Or, on the other hand, he may take the news badly and arrange to meet with a solicitor to make his will. But no matter how he acts, it may be legitimately asked whether he would feel any differently if he were told that the risk was 6% or 8%? Would he really be able to convince us that there was a difference? And if there was no difference between his attitude to 7% and that to 6%, then what would the information that a drug reduces mortality from 7% to 6% mean to him? Surely, in these circumstances, it would be as reasonable – if not, indeed, more reasonable - to decline long-term treatment as to accept it. Of course, it might be argued that the important point is that the risk is reduced but this is also true when the drug reduces mortality from 0.7% to 0.6% and few would argue that the latter results would support the use of long-term drug therapy. (For further discussion, see Chapter V.)

A clearer perspective may be gained by considering the proportion of patients who obtain no benefit from the treatment. The only reliable generalisation that may be derived from mega-trials is that the drug has no beneficial effect on the vast majority of the study population. For example, according to the LIPID study[19], the CARE study[20] and the GISSI-3 study[12], more than 98% of patients who are prescribed the drug will not only derive no advantage but will be subjected to possible adverse-effects. In this context, it is worth remembering the recent withdrawal of cerivastatin: in all probability, those patients who died from the side-effects were receiving this drug with little prospect of obtaining benefit.

Mega-trials (Data for Primary Endpoints)			
	Outcome	Absolute Reduction	Patients with no benefit
LIPID study[19]	Mortality	1.9%	98.1%
CARE study[20]	Stroke	1.2%	98.8%
HOPE study[18]	Composite	3.8%	96.2%
GISSI-3 study[12]	Composite	1.4%	98.6%
ISIS-2 study[14]	Mortality	2.8%	97.2%

The issue of small treatment effects has recently been addressed by Freemantle and Hill,[22] also using the example of long-term therapy with statins, who remarked that *"Rich western societies are investing in preventative treatments that will benefit only a minority of those who take them for a long time."* Noting that these drugs were now taken regularly by more than 5% of the entire population of the United States and acknowledging that more than 97.5% of patients receiving statins for five years derive no benefit, they argued that *"The increasing number of patients included in the clinical trials of statins bears testament to the increasingly small treatment effects that are of interest."*

The crux of the problem is that the meaning of small differences is unclear. As such, they are unable to offer any firm guide to action, either on the part of an individual patient or on the part of the doctor involved in their care.

Small treatment effects and populations

While the case in favour of using drugs based on the results of mega-trials is difficult to sustain in the individual patient, the problem of a small treatment difference appears less important when considered in the context of large populations of patients. In other words, while a small treatment difference may offer little benefit to an individual patient, it is claimed that the widespread use of the drug in a common disease would prevent morbidity and mortality in many thousands of patients. However, despite the support generated by intricate calculations estimating the potential number of lives that would be saved and by detailed cost-benefit analyses, this argument does not stand up to scrutiny.

Nothing in the population approach negates the potential for error in the assessment of internal validity. Similarly, nothing addresses the problem of causal inference. And nothing inflates the paltry difference in outcome among the treatment groups. But even if these problems are disregarded, the limitations in external validity compromise any claim of benefit in the wider population. The selection criteria as well as participation in the study militate against any reliable generalisation. Given the small subgroup of patients involved in the treatment effect, it is easy to conceive of circumstances in which this proportion might change in such a way that the reported benefit would no longer be present. Moreover, the possible adverse effects of treatment may be more pronounced in patients excluded from the study, thus further lessening the overall benefit were the drug to be widely prescribed.

In any case, even if the only problem associated with mega-trials were to be the small treatment effect, the argument that a drug should be used because of the benefits to the wider population would be unacceptable. Once it is acknowledged that the small treatment effect offers little benefit to any individual, the possible benefits to the wider population are not relevant to any decision that a doctor might take about any particular patient. If there is little prospect of a patient gaining any benefit from the drug, then it should not be prescribed. To do otherwise, would be to put the interest of the patient second behind that of the wider community.

Whenever any treatment is recommended on the basis of results from a mega-trial, it is important to distinguish between arguments in favour of its use in individuals and in populations. Yet, this distinction is rarely made. Instead, the two aspects are blurred: the weaknesses of the argument in individuals are assumed to be counteracted by the strengths of the argument in populations and vice versa. Once separated, however, it becomes clear that each argument has to stand alone. In particular, if the argument in favour of treatment in individuals fails, then that is an end to the matter, regardless of any possible benefits in the wider population.

Replication and Mega-trials

As discussed earlier, replication is a cardinal feature of the scientific method. The precision of the definitions of materials and methods permits an accurate specification of the conditions of an experiment, thus enabling other researchers to recreate the identical conditions in order to test the original findings. In these circumstances, any discrepancy between the results raises serious questions about the original study.

When, however, it comes to mega-trials, the case is very different. Given the inability to specify accurately the study population in terms of all relevant variables, any attempt at replication will be open to challenge. If a further study fails to show the same effect as the original, it may be dismissed on the grounds that the study populations were different. But, if replication cannot falsify the results of the original study, then neither can it confirm the results. For, if a study is to confirm the results of another, the initial conditions must be the same; yet this is precisely what is rejected when replication fails. Known or unknown differences in the distribution of relevant variables among study populations makes each mega-trial unique and, hence, their results are not strictly comparable. All that remains is to tolerate a series of inconsistent results. It is hardly surprising, therefore, that reviews in the medical literature frequently include randomised trials with inconsistent findings.

The absence of replication in mega-trials is of the utmost importance. It greatly lessens the reliability of the results, it removes a primary method of avoiding fraud and it prevents any check on the validity of the methodology.

Mega-trials - Science or an Alternative Methodology?

Science is characterised by the quest for knowledge of the natural world. A scientific theory is judged in accordance with its success in predicting events in the world around us. The aim of science is to provide accurate and reliable generalisations which may be used for practical purposes. And the results are everywhere around us: the construction of buildings and bridges; the delivery of heating and light to our homes; transport by car, train and aeroplane; clean water at the turn of a tap, food surviving months in the freezer, instant hot meals from the microwave; entertainment from radio, television and CD player; communication across continents at the touch of a mobile phone button; computers, satellites.... The list is endless. We are immersed in a world teeming with proof of the success of science.

The scientific method delivers reliable generalisations in the form of universal propositions attributing a particular characteristic to all members of the reference class. As emphasized repeatedly, it is the existence of sound background theory which is crucial to the success of science. It is the framework against which observations are made, it allows strict definition of the items involved, it is the source of information about possible relevant variables and allows for the identification of homogeneous reference classes that ensure regularity and, hence, reliable causal inference. Furthermore, in line with the requirement for a body of knowledge to contain only logically consistent premises, the background theory regulates which generalisations may be accepted, thus providing a further check on the validity of new findings. Finally, the generalisations may readily be confirmed by replication.

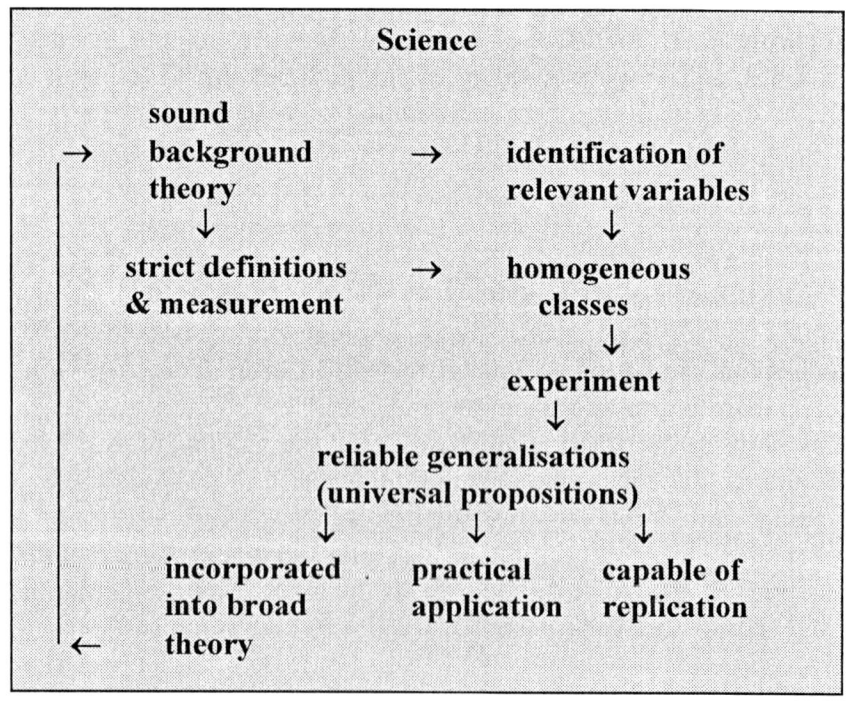

The contrast with mega-trials in medical research could not be more obvious. Without sound background theory and knowledge, heterogeneous classes are, in most clinical situations, unavoidable. The proposed solution to this problem – randomisation - fails in practice to deliver internal validity. Mega-trials also suffer from intractable problems in terms of external validity. Moreover, not only are the small treatment effects undetectable in routine clinical practice but there is no prospect of confirmation by replication.

These considerations raise a fundamental question: what is the justification for the methodology of mega-trials? The usual answer would be that mega-trials involve the use of the scientific method, albeit with minor alterations, and that since the scientific method has proved itself over hundreds of years, no further justification is required for mega-trials. Such arguments, however, are difficult to reconcile with the clear differences between the experiments of science and clinical research involving large-scale randomised controlled trials.

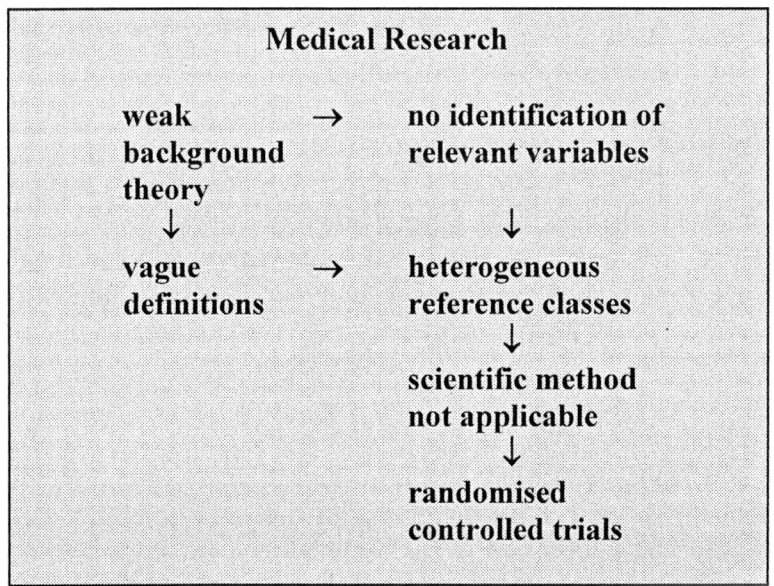

If mega-trials are not grounded in the scientific method, then the only alternative would be to view them as an entirely different approach to the identification of causal relationships in the natural world. Accordingly, mega-trials would be distinct from the scientific method and their methodology would stand alone. But then, of course, this prompts the question of whether or not the methodology is valid. Just as in the case of the scientific method, mega-trials would have to prove their worth. And this is precisely were the difficulty lies. No individual instance could verify the conclusion of a mega-trial. Furthermore, no series of individual instances in routine clinical practice could verify its conclusion. And, while it may be claimed that the results of other mega-trials validate the conclusion, this is not the case. A further study with conflicting results would not be accepted as a refutation of the original mega-trial since differences in the study populations, in the definitions of disease, in the precise treatment regimen and in many other respects would be invoked to explain the different outcomes. But, if studies with conflicting data cannot refute the original results, then studies with similar results cannot confirm them. Thus, if the mega-trial does stand alone, then it is exposed to the charge that since its results cannot be confirmed they are, therefore, without foundation.

Conclusions

All randomised trials regardless of the number of patients involved, are subject to the pitfalls of faulty randomisation, inadequate blinding and errors in the analysis of data that jeopardise internal validity, as well as to the ever-present threats to external validity. However, large-scale randomised trials suffer from additional problems that stem from the fundamental features of these studies.

The small treatment differences, which are the inevitable product of mega-trials, have major implications. They aggravate the uncertainties already present in randomised trials in respect of both internal and external validity. In the context of an individual patient, a small treatment difference entails only a remote chance of benefit; indeed, the vast majority of patients will receive treatment unnecessarily whilst being exposed to adverse drug reactions, often for long periods of time. Claims that treatment based on small differences may be justified in terms of the benefits to be expected from the use of the drug in the wider population of patients are not sustainable given the problems with external validity that are endemic in mega-trials.

Of even greater concern than the small differences is the lack of any firm foundation for the methodology. Any comparison of mega-trials with science reveals that they are fundamentally different. On the one hand, science is characterised by strong background theory that allows the formation of homogeneous reference classes which, in turn, yield reliable generalisations with definite practical applications. Mega-trials, on the other hand, deal with heterogeneous classes with all the ensuing challenges to internal and external validity. The scientific method is founded on the principles of induction and causation, whereas mega-trials, eschewing the requirements for resemblance and regularity, rely instead on the statistical notion of causation. Given the extent of these differences, the methodology of mega-trials cannot be grounded in the scientific method. Science is of proven value; its successes are everywhere to be seen; any doubts may easily be dispelled by the observation of individual instances of the phenomenon or, more formally, by replication. These options, though, are not available to mega-trials. If, as is argued, they are distinct from science, then they must stand alone and demonstrate their validity independently. But how is this to be achieved? In the absence of a satisfactory reply, the results of mega-trials must remain in limbo.

References

1. Koch R. *Ueber bakteriologische Forschung.* Veh X. Int Med Congr Berlin, 1890. P35; 1892.

2. Surgeon General's Advisory Committee on Smoking and Health . US Department of Health, Education & Welfare; 1103; Chap 3. 1964.

3. Hill AB. The environment and disease: association or causation? *Proc Roy Soc Med* 1965; 58;295-300.

4. Feinstein AR. Scientific standards vs. statistical associations and biologic logic in the analysis of causation. *Clin Pharmacol Ther* 1979;25;481-92.

5. Susser M. Rules of inference in epidemiology. *Reg Toxicol Pharmacol* 1986;6;116-28.

6. Doll R, Hill AB. Mortality in relation to smoking: Ten years' observations of British doctors. *Br Med J* 1964;i;1399-1410.

7. Snow J. *On the Mode of Communication of Cholera.* London, 1855.

8. Susser M. Falsification, verification and causal inference in epidemiology: reconsiderations in the light of Sir Karl Popper's philosophy. In: *Causal Inference.* Edited by KJ Rothman. Epidemiology Resources Inc. 1988. Pages 33-58.

9. Leibovici L. Effects of remote, retroactive intercessory prayer on outcomes in patients with bloodstream infections: randomised controlled trial. *Br Med J* 2001;323;1450-1.

10. ASSET study group. Trial of tissue plasminogen activator for mortality reduction in acute myocardial infarction. Anglo-Scandinavian Study of Early Thrombolysis (ASSET). *Lancet* 1988;ii;525-30.

11. Gruppo Italiano per lo Studio della Sopravvivenza nell'Infarcto Miocardico. GISSI-2: a factorial randomised trial of alteplase versus streptokinase and heparin versus no heparin among 12,490 patients with acute myocardial infarction. *Lancet* 1990;336;65-71.

12. Gruppo Italiano per lo Studio della Sopravvivenza nell'Infarcto Miocardico. GISSI-3: effects of lisinopril and transdermal glyceryl trinitrate singly and together on 6-week mortality and ventricular function after acute myocardial infarction. *Lancet* 1994;343;1115-22.

13. LATE Study Group. Late assessment of thrombolytic efficacy (LATE) study with alteplase 6-24 hours after onset of acute myocardial infarction. *Lancet* 1993;342;759-66.

14. ISIS-2 (Second International Study of Infarct Survival) Collaborative Group. Randomised trial of intravenous streptokinase, oral aspirin, both or neither among 17187 cases of suspected acute myocardial infarction: ISIS-2. *Lancet* 1988;2;349-60.

15. ISIS-3 (Third International Study of Infarct Survival) Collaborative Group. ISIS-3: a randomised comparison of streptokinase vs tissue plasminogen activator vs anistreplase and of aspirin plus heparin vs aspirin alone among 41,299 cases of suspected acute myocardial infarction. *Lancet* 1992;339;753-70.

16. Assessment of the Safety and Efficacy of a New Thrombolytic (ASSENT-2) Investigators. Single-bolus tenecteplase compared with front-loaded alteplase in acute myocardial infarction: the ASSENT-2 double-blind randomised trial. *Lancet* 1999;354;716-22.

17. Dixon G, Boyle RM, Norris RM. Clinical trials in acute myocardial infarction versus real life: a limitation of evidence-based medicine. *Br J Cardiol* 2000;7;709-11.

18. The Heart Outcomes Prevention Evaluation Study Investigators. Effects of an angiotensin-converting-enzyme inhibitor, ramipril, on cardiovascular events in high-risk patients. *New Eng J Med* 2000;342;145-153.

19. The Long-Term Intervention with Pravastatin in Ischaemic Disease (LIPID) Study Group. Prevention of cardiovascular events and death with pravastatin in patients with coronary heart disease and a broad range of initial cholesterol levels. *New Eng J Med* 1998;339;1349-57.

20. Plehn JF, Davis BR, Sacks FM, et al. Reduction of stroke incidence after myocardial infarction with pravastatin. . The Cholesterol and Recurrent Events (CARE) Study. *Circulation* 1999;99;216-23.

21. Edwards A, Elwyn G, Mulley A. Explaining risks: turning numerical data into meaningful pictures. *Br Med J* 2002;324;827-30.

22. Freemantle N & Hill S. Medicalisation, limits to medicine, or never enough money to go around? *Br Med J* 2002;324;864-5.

V

THE FALL-OUT FROM FAULTY SCIENCE

If the use of mega-trials were confined to the investigation of some esoteric subdivision of North Sea algae or the mating rituals of a rare species of South American spider, then we could safely ignore the entire enterprise. The problem, of course, is that these studies have an enormous impact on the lives of millions of patients throughout the world. Whether or not they offer any genuine benefits is debatable. Certainly, the methodology is so clearly flawed that any claim that they improve the lives of those suffering from the common chronic diseases must be viewed with the utmost suspicion.

But, setting aside the methodological failings, it becomes clear that mega-trials raise other important issues in relation to medical research. Are the data, for instance, sufficiently robust to withstand attempts at manipulation? Or, instead, are they so loose as to allow a free interpretation by those with a vested interest in the outcome? Do mega-trials offer any substantial defence against fraud? Are treatments based on these studies a waste of health-care resources? And what are the ethical implications of recommending treatment supported by the results of mega-trials?

Manipulation of Data

Large-scale randomised trials are highly complex processes and the published studies are both lengthy and detailed. Given the thousands of words of text, together with an array of tables and figures, the data are rarely transparent. An accurate appraisal of these papers requires many hours of study and is really only accessible to those who are both conversant with the methodology and who have specialist knowledge of the subject involved.

The unwieldy nature of mega-trials and their opaque content, particularly when considered in the context of both the widespread uncertainties in the methodology and the small treatment differences, allow a great deal of latitude in the interpretation of their results. These features also tend to disguise the manipulation of data frequently present.

Inflating small treatment effects

The current fashion for reporting the results of mega-trials in terms of the relative risk reduction speaks volumes for the trivial nature of the absolute difference. At a stroke, it converts small differences into something apparently more clinically relevant. The practice of emphasizing the relative risk reduction while paying scant attention to the absolute risk reduction is misleading because it creates the illusion of a substantial difference.

Any reduction in relative risk must be interpreted in the context of the reduction in absolute risk. This requirement is clearly shown by the following example in which the relative risk reduction remains constant while the absolute risk reduction varies from a valuable treatment effect to a clinically irrelevant difference.

Mortality		Relative Risk	Absolute Risk
Placebo	Drug	Reduction	Reduction
80%	60%	25%	20%
8%	6%	25%	2%
0.8%	0.6%	25%	0.2%

The relative risk reduction, as opposed to the absolute risk reduction, concerns only a subgroup of the study population. This may be seen from the way in which the relative risk reduction is calculated: if n_1 and n_2 are the numbers of patients dying in the placebo and active treatment groups respectively, and since the two groups are randomly allocated they will effectively have the same number of patients (N), then the relative risk reduction is $[(n_1/N - n_2/N)/(n_1/N)]$ which, simplified, becomes $[(n_1 - n_2)/n_1]$. In other words, reference to the study population is cancelled out leaving the relative risk reduction relating only to a small subgroup of patients developing the outcome.

The absolute difference between the placebo and treatment groups is the most informative measure of the benefit of the drug under investigation. Unlike the relative risk reduction, the absolute risk reduction $[(n_1 - n_2)/N]$ maintains the link to the study population thereby avoiding any misleading interpretation. Large reductions in the absolute risk have obvious clinical importance. However, mega-trials yield only small differences which are of debatable value and it is essential that this crucial aspect is not hidden beneath the advertising headlines based on relative risk reductions.

Misleading Relative Risk Reductions		
	Mortality	
	Relative Reduction	Absolute Reduction
ASSET study[1]	26%	2.6%
ISIS-2 study[2]	25%	2.8%
GUSTO study[3]	14%	1%
GISSI-3 study[4]	11%	0.8%
HOPE study[5]	16%	1.8%

The use of relative risk reductions is nowadays a common feature of studies in the medical literature. In the field of cardiovascular disease, where mega-trials are ubiquitous, it is not difficult to find examples of studies emphasizing the relative risk reduction.[1-5] Such reports give a false impression of the size of the benefit from a particular treatment which is not, however, present when attention is focussed on the absolute risk reduction. Moreover, the presentation of relative risk reductions while avoiding mention of the absolute differences in the abstract is a frequent practice that deliberately misleads those readers who have little time to study the entire paper.

Although the trend for focussing on relative risks has been criticised,[6,7] the practice is widespread.[8] This is hardly surprising, given the benefit of reporting this statistic to those involved in the promotion of new treatments.[9] Clearly, the way in which the results are presented affects the therapeutic decisions made by doctors and health authorities.[10,11] For example, the use of relative risk reductions has been shown to produce a falsely high impression of the treatment effect.[12,13]

It is easy to see why the relative risk reduction is a popular measure of the outcome in mega-trials. It provides a more impressive headline figure for the investigators to include in their publication and allows those funding the study to make exaggerated claims for their drug. This emphasis, however, may have a more insidious effect in that, by obscuring the small absolute difference, it lessens the awareness of the flaws and inhibits criticism of the methodology of mega-trials.

The use of the relative risk reduction is tantamount to a statistical sleight of hand disguising the trivial nature of the treatment difference in large-scale randomised trials.

Exaggerated conclusions of mega-trials

The complexity and vagueness of the data of mega-trials, together with an absence of any incontrovertible and observable effect, obscure the exaggerations frequently present in the conclusions.

The LIPID study[14], for example, investigated the effect of pravastatin in 9014 patients with established ischaemic heart disease. During an observation period of six years, the overall mortality was11% in the pravastatin group compared with 14.1% in those receiving placebo, the absolute difference in mortality being 3.1%. These results, of course, reflect the presence of heterogeneity in both the pravastatin and placebo groups which, in turn, expose the weaknesses of the underlying theory – in particular, the uncertainties of the link between alterations in blood lipids and future cardiovascular events, as well as ignorance of the other relevant variables involved in the outcome. On the basis of the LIPID study[14], the authors surprisingly claimed that *"Because of our results, cholesterol-lowering therapy should now be considered for virtually all patients presenting with CHD"*. But, given the small treatment differences and the questionable background knowledge, is such a conclusion really justified? Surely, the best that may be said for the results is that they suggest that there is small, unspecified group of patients with heart disease who are likely to die during a follow-up period of six years and that one-fifth of this group may survive because of treatment with cholesterol-lowering drugs.

A further example of the exaggerated conclusions of mega-trials may be observed in the CARE study[15] which reported the effect of pravastatin on the subsequent development of strokes during five years after myocardial infarction. Based on a relative risk reduction in stroke of 32%, the authors claimed that the results *"...established the value of lipid modification with pravastatin in reducing stroke..."*. However, even a brief examination of the paper raises questions about this conclusion. The 95% confidence intervals for the relative risk reduction in stroke were wide (4% to 52%) and the P-value only just reached statistical significance (P = 0.03). More importantly, the absolute difference in the rate of stroke between placebo and pravastatin was a mere 1.2%. Once again, the results draw attention to the presence of heterogeneity and limited background theory – on this occasion, the authors explicitly acknowledged the uncertainties concerning the link between cholesterol reduction and the development of strokes. In addition, whilst the authors expected a reduction specifically in ischaemic stroke, as opposed to haemorrhagic cerebro-vascular events, this was not present, thus further challenging the background theory. After studying more than 4000 patients for five years, all that was found was a barely significant difference between placebo and pravastatin in terms of overall strokes, and no significant difference in the occurrence of ischaemic strokes. Taken in conjunction with the conflicting background evidence, are the results of this study really all that it takes to establish a new treatment?

The standard of evidence supporting the use of statins in these studies is highly questionable yet 11.5 million patients in the United States take this medication every day on the basis of dubious data and exaggerated conclusions in the published studies.[16] While certainly not confined to therapy with statins, exaggerating the data from mega-trials assists in the marketing of a new drug and results in its widespread but unwarranted use.

Excessive latitude allowing free interpretation of data

At first sight, the National Institute for Clinical Excellence established by the government in 1999 appears to be a promising advance in the delivery of health care. It is designed to assess new treatments and make recommendations concerning their use within the NHS, thus promoting uniform health care of a high standard across England and Wales. An appraisal committee appointed for three years, supplemented by experts in the relevant field of medicine, reaches a decision on the basis of the evidence available. NICE, it seems, has all the attributes required to ensure wise judgments. But when tested, it has been shown to be defective.

In October 1999, NICE reported on a new drug for the treatment of influenza.[17] The conclusion - that zanamivir should not be prescribed - proved to be controversial. Glaxo Wellcome, the manufacturers of zanamivir, were reported to have reacted to the decision by threatening to transfer their research outside of the United Kingdom. Yet NICE had based its decision on the results of clinical trials and was fully supported by an independent, comprehensive review of the subject.[18] Only one year later, however, NICE had reversed its decision in respect of a subgroup of patients suffering from influenza.[19]

This remarkable *volte-face* says a great deal both about NICE and about the data on which its decision was reached. According to the most recent communication relating to zanamivir,[19] NICE considered eleven randomised controlled trials involving more than 3000 patients and pooled the results. The analysis showed that, compared to placebo, the drug reduced the duration of symptoms from six to five days. Such trivial findings justified the original conclusion by NICE that zanamivir should not be used in patients with influenza. Attention then turned to patients at particular risk from influenza. A separate analysis of approximately 800 "at-risk" patients again showed that zanamivir reduced the duration of symptoms by one day, although the upper 95% confidence interval was close to zero. More importantly, whilst the drug was reported to reduce the risk of complications requiring antibiotics, the absolute reduction was a mere 6% with 95% confidence intervals of 0% to 11%. Given this very small difference and its borderline statistical significance, together with the fact that no data were available in relation to the effect of the drug on either the rate of complications requiring admission to hospital or on mortality, the conclusion by NICE that zanamivir should be recommended for at-risk adults appears perverse.

There are also further reasons to question the use of zanamivir in routine clinical practice. As noted in the review in the *Drug and Therapeutics Bulletin*, [18] the availability of the drug only on prescription entails that patients have to visit their general practitioner but such behaviour is not consistent with the general advice in the context of influenza to stay at home and avoid further spread of the disease; moreover, it would place increasing demands on general practitioners during influenza outbreaks. Other problems arise from the specific indications recommended by NICE: if treatment is only to be given to patients presenting within 36 hours of the onset of symptoms, individuals who believe the drug will be of benefit may be inclined to report a shorter duration of symptoms than is otherwise the case in order to ensure receiving the medication; and, when under pressure from patients for the "new" treatment for influenza, general practitioners may well attempt to avoid confrontation by relaxing the criteria for "at-risk" groups. Finally, uncertainty remains concerning the frequency with which resistance develops to zanamivir.

In the face of the inadequate evidence of efficacy and the potential adverse consequences, it is difficult to avoid the suspicion that the recent guidance from NICE relating to zanamivir was influenced either by political considerations or by the vested interests of the pharmaceutical industry. Whatever the true reasons, the reputation of NICE has been tarnished. Glossy brochures will not be enough to rid the National Institute for Clinical Excellence of the lingering doubts about its objectivity and impartiality.

But laying the blame for the zanamivir episode exclusively at the door of NICE is to miss a crucial aspect of the affair. The results of clinical trials allowed NICE such a degree of latitude in their interpretation of the data that they were able to reach any decision they desired and still claim that it was consistent with the evidence. The paltry differences in the outcomes could have been rejected on the grounds that they had no clinical importance; alternatively, given that they were statistically significant, the results could have been used to support a recommendation for zanamivir to be made widely available for the treatment of influenza. This confusion was present whether NICE was considering results for the overall population of patients with influenza or for those relating to the "at-risk" groups. In fact, the statistical analysis was less robust in the latter setting, making the change of policy even more suspect.

As long as medical research persists with clinical trials which yield trivial differences, the results will remain open to manipulation. Moreover, as long as NICE continues to entertain such faulty research - instead of rejecting it outright - it will be handed one poisoned chalice after another until it consumes one draft too many. The National Institute for Clinical Excellence would surely have won plaudits if it had used common sense and, after examining the evidence for zanamivir, had proclaimed the drug to be a waste of scarce health care resources. But instead, it jettisoned its integrity and succumbed to the lethal cocktail of the sophistry of randomised trials and the influence of vested interests from politics and the pharmaceutical industry.

Misleading conclusions from mega-trials

There is an even more serious aspect to the reporting of mega-trials that involves conclusions which are not consistent with the actual data relating to the study. Consider, for example, the GISSI-3 study[4] which compared the effects of lisinopril, nitrates, both treatments or placebo in more than 19,000 patients with acute myocardial infarction. An initial examination of the data reveals the usual problems encountered in all mega-trials. For example, the exclusion of 55% of the patients with myocardial infarction greatly limited the external validity of the results. Furthermore, the treatment differences were very small. These features of the trial, however, did not inhibit the authors from concluding: *"Lisinopril produced significant reductions in overall mortality and in the combined outcome measure of mortality and severe ventricular dysfunction"*. These claims were based on a comparison between lisinopril (with or without nitrates) and "controls" (which comprised patients receiving either placebo or nitrates alone). According to this analysis, the absolute difference in mortality between lisinopril and controls was 0.8% and that in the combined endpoint of mortality plus left ventricular dysfunction was 1.4%. Such trivial treatment differences and highly questionable external validity are the standard fare of mega-trials, thus making the conclusion unexceptional in this context.

However, there is a further aspect which militates against the authors' conclusion. The GISSI-3 study[4] also reported data which showed that when lisinopril alone was compared with placebo alone, the absolute differences in overall mortality and in the combined endpoint were each 0.6%, neither result being statistically significant. In other words, a direct comparison between lisinopril and placebo in more than 9,000 patients demonstrated no difference in outcome – a finding that contradicts the authors' conclusion. How did this unsatisfactory state of affairs arise?

GISSI-3 Study[4]		
	Mortality	Combined Endpoint
Overall Analysis		
Controls (placebo or nitrates)	7.1%	17.0%
v		
Lisinopril (+/- nitrates)	6.3%	15.6%
Specific comparison		
Placebo alone	7.2%	17.0%
v		
Lisinopril alone	6.6%	16.4%

The publication of this misleading conclusion stems from a variety of sources. The complexity of the data in the GISSI-3 study, as in all mega-trials, makes a detailed appraisal difficult and time-consuming. This, presumably, accounts for the failure of the peer review process in this study. But what about the responsibility of the investigators? Surely some of the hundreds of researchers listed at the end of the paper would have drawn attention to this error? The decision to use only data from the overall results in the abstract – while avoiding the direct comparison of lisinopril with placebo – indicates how the presentation of data may be manipulated in mega-trials. This is clearly to the advantage of those with a vested interest in the outcome. In this regard, it is to be noted that the study was supported by the manufacturers of lisinopril.

The GISSI-3 study shows just how easy it is to manipulate the results of mega-trials in support of the desired outcome and to hide these distortions amongst a mass of data. As with the reporting of most mega-trials, the GISSI-3 study[4] published in the *Lancet* is opaque. Large amounts of data are crammed into paragraphs, tables and figures. It takes a considerable time to digest all the detailed information and even longer to dissect out the errors. And, as in the case of other mega-trials, what is reported in the abstract is not necessarily an accurate reflection of what is contained in the paper.

No Protection against Vested Interests

Inflated results, exaggerated conclusions, interpretations divorced from the actual data, and false claims all stem from the nature of mega-trials. The weaknesses of this methodology allow – if not, indeed, encourage - those with a vested interest in the outcome of mega-trials to use the data for their own advantage. In other words, the complexity and vagueness of mega-trials, the small treatment differences and the lack of any observable effects provide ample scope for arguing in favour of a variety of opposing positions.

Those with a vested interest in the results of mega-trials include medical researchers, patient-groups, the National Health Service management, government and, of course the pharmaceutical industry.[20,21] Frequently, the various groups interact. For example, it is well recognised that there is disturbing conflict of interest between medical researchers and the pharmaceutical industry.[21] A recent study investigating the relationship between the conclusions of studies and the financial interests of the investigators in 159 randomised clinical trials reported that the authors' conclusions favoured a treatment effect in trials funded by the pharmaceutical industry. [22] These findings are supported by other studies.[23] It is hardly surprising that the pharmaceutical industry has a large influence on medical researchers. In the past, many clinical trials have been sponsored by the private sector and this trend appears to be increasing.[24] Those involved in medical research often have financial ties with industry in the form of payments for patients recruited to the studies, fees for lecturing, support for attendance at meetings and funding for their departments. In the circumstances, it is only to be expected that the conclusions of the studies will tend to reflect well on the pharmaceutical company while any unfavourable data such as side-effects will be played down[25] if not, indeed, deliberately suppressed.[21]

The effect of vested interests on the decisions of the National Institute of Clinical Excellence regarding zanamivir remains shrouded in mystery. Was the original recommendation to reject the drug affected by political considerations? And was the subsequent change of heart influenced by the pharmaceutical company? Similar uncertainties surround the Institute's recommendations concerning imatinib, a new drug for the treatment of chronic myeloid leukaemia. However, NICE is not alone in being open to manipulation. The influence of the pharmaceutical industry on government institutions and regularity authorities is of general concern, particularly as the latter are often dependent upon funding received from pharmaceutical companies.[20]

The United States Food and Drug Administration has also been involved in a startling about-turn. Alosetron (Lotronex) was approved by the FDA for use in patients with irritable bowel syndrome in February 2000. While the manufacturers, GlaxoSmithKline, described the drug as "highly efficacious", the FDA recognised only "modest benefits" and others considered the claims by the investigators to be greatly exaggerated with only marginal advantages over placebo.[26] Following reports of serious adverse drug reactions – in particular, severe constipation requiring hospitalisation or surgery and cases of ischaemic colitis – approval was withdrawn later the same year. By April 2002, alosetron was believed to be responsible for more than 100 hospital admissions, 50 patients requiring surgical procedures and seven deaths. Despite the mounting casualties, a few months later, the FDA approved the use of alosetron in women with diarrhoea-predominant irritable bowel syndrome.[26] Was this move the result of publicity generated by the Lotronex Action Group which lobbies on behalf of patients with irritable bowel syndrome and is sponsored by GlaxoSmithKline?[27] Or was it direct pressure from the pharmaceutical industry which provides much of the funding for the FDA? When a regulatory authority – especially one as prestigious as the FDA – succumbs to the demands of the pharmaceutical industry and approves the use of a drug with marginal benefits for a benign, mostly trivial disease in the face of numerous reports of serious adverse reactions to that drug, the alarm bells should ring.

Away from government creations like the FDA and NICE, it might be assumed that a more neutral appraisal of new drugs would be provided by institutions within medicine itself. Regrettably, this does not appear to be the case. The recently issued guidelines by the American Heart Association recommending the widespread use of thrombolytic drugs for patients with strokes has again raised serious questions about conflict of interest.[28] In a comprehensive account in the *British Medical Journal*,[29] Lenzer exposed the financial links between Genentech, the manufacturers of alteplase, and the American Heart Association. Over the past decade, the American Heart Association has received $11m from Genentech and six of the nine members of the panel drawing up the guidelines had financial ties with the company. In the light of these revelations, the impartiality of the guidelines is clearly brought into question. Once again, though, a biased interpretation of the data would not be possible were the results of the clinical trials uncontroversial. Whilst some interpret the data as convincing evidence of benefit,[28,30] others consider that the case for alteplase in stroke has yet to be established.[31-33]   Lenzer, however, presents a cogent argument against the position adopted by the American Heart Association.[29] The guidelines were based primarily on the National Institute of Neurological Diseases and Stroke study[34] which has been criticised on the grounds of baseline imbalance, questionable external validity and a marginal therapeutic benefit from alteplase; data from other studies showing an increased mortality in stroke patients receiving thrombolysis were ignored; Genentech refused access to the raw data of the relevant clinical trials; and, finally, claims by the American Heart Association that alteplase saved lives in patients with stroke were later withdrawn.[29]

The influence of the pharmaceutical industry and other groups with a vested interest in the results of clinical trials is nothing new. As the above examples show, institutions founded either by government, such as the FDA and NICE, or by the medical profession, such as the American Heart Association, are not immune to these influences. Despite an increasing awareness of conflicts of interest and proposals to address these problems,[35] it is likely that the manipulation of results and the incorrect recommendations for treatment will continue as long as the quality of the data from clinical trials remains poor. In this context, large-scale randomised trials are even more susceptible to manipulation and distortion of data than are the medium-sized studies related to zanamivir, alosetron and alteplase. The very small treatment effects characteristic of mega-trials allow even greater scope for biased interpretation.

Bringing Medical Research into Disrepute

Nowadays, it seems that no edition of a newspaper is complete without a medical scare story. And the hundreds of medical journals offer an ample source of dubious associations between environmental exposure and disease. Many of these reports are based on observational studies, the limitations of which are seldom appreciated by the medical profession, let alone by the lay public. Adding salt to meals, drinking coffee, using mobile phones, living in close proximity to electricity pylons and receiving the MMR vaccine have all been linked to various diseases over recent years without any firm evidence, leading to unnecessary concern and worry amongst the general public. Although the standard of reporting of medical issues in the lay press contributes to the misunderstandings,[36] the ensuing disputes amongst members of the medical profession create the impression of utter confusion and engender a sceptical approach to medical research.

Whilst it is generally assumed that randomised controlled trials deliver reliable data on which to base decisions concerning the management of patients, the methodology has done little to avoid the clash of opinions in the medical journals and the lay press. The skirmishes relating to thrombolytic therapy in patients with stroke[29-33] are typical and have already been discussed. Even when considering large-scale randomised trials, controversy still exists, as, for example, in the case of long-term aspirin therapy following myocardial infarction.[37-39] A further example relates to screening for breast cancer: although hundreds of thousands of women have been recruited to large-scale trials, arguments continue to rage over the value of mammography.[40-42] Indeed, so polarised has this argument become, that it prompted the editor of the Lancet to describe a recent exchange on the subject as: *"Two different reviews in two separate journals, together with confusion, anger, recrimination, bitterness, and a private e-mail exchange that deserves publication in its own right as a study in the socio(patho)logy of science."* [43] It is not difficult to understand the present disenchantment with medical research.[35] The frequent disputes that are aired in journals spill over into the national press bringing the whole of medical research into disrepute. The solution, however, is not to attempt to suppress argument[43] but, instead, to address the origin of the problem, *viz.* the failure of the large scale randomised trials – the "gold standard" in medical research - to deliver reliable generalisations.

No Defence against Fraud

Regardless of how meticulous the efforts are to create a secure scientific method, all research is open to fraud. In *Betrayers of the Truth* (1985), Broad and Wade provided a comprehensive account of fraud across a variety of scientific disciplines.[44] They described a spectrum of offences - from the minor manipulation of data and plagiarism to the fabrication of entire research studies - throughout the history of science involving offenders as famous as Ptolemy, Newton, Dalton and Mendel.

Fraud occurs because of a failure of the normal mechanisms to ensure that research is properly conducted together with the dishonesty of individual researchers.[44] The first protection against fraud is the supervision by heads of departments; this may, of course range from a diligent, watchful eye on their junior staff to a complete abandonment of responsibility. The approval of referees before publication is considered an essential part of the assessment of research but it must not be forgotton than referees not only vary in their quality but have, almost by necessity, an interest either in the acceptance or the rejection of the findings; hence the selection of referees by the editors of journals plays a major role in determining whether or not the work is published. Once in print, further judgment on the study depends on scrutiny by the scientific community; this, in turn, depends to a large extent on an examination of the raw data which may not be available in the publication. The final arbiter of the validity of research is replication of the experiment.

The prevalence of fraud in medicine is unknown although Broad and Wade document many examples as well as drawing attention to the particular circumstances in which medical research is conducted.[44] Experience in research and the acquisition of an M.D. Thesis are often viewed as no more than a chore to be endured in order to increase the prospects of a consultant appointment. Research, as Broad and Wade remark, is not so much a vocation as a stepping stone to progress in a non-research career. One or two years of research may yield the desired paper qualification but it is unlikely to produce work of any quality, while the pressures to complete the studies in a limited amount of time will encourage some to engage in fraudulent activities.

Unfortunately, unlike most scientific disciplines in which fraud may be readily detected by attempts at replication, the special circumstances surrounding mega-trials preclude this crucial check on the validity of research. The complexity and opaque nature of large-scale trials, the small treatment differences amenable to manipulation, the enormous potential profits for a successful new drug in common chronic diseases and the whole enterprise under the influence of those with vested interests in the outcome are fertile ground for fraud. But, most crucial of all is the strong likelihood that the fraud will remain undetected. Observations made in routine clinical practice will never be sufficient to disprove the results of a mega-trial, while replication is weakened to such an extent that it no longer has the power to discriminate between authentic and flawed research.

In a recent leading article in the *British Medical Journal*, Farthing et al.[45] commented on the failure of the medical establishment to address the problem of fraud. They noted that the Royal College of Physicians of London had published a report[46] on research fraud a decade ago yet this had been ignored. Moreover, they were critical that, despite the Edinburgh conference[47] in 2000 recognising that fraud in medical research was a problem, nothing had been done to begin implementing the recommendations. Increasingly, fraud is being recognised as presenting a serious threat to the integrity of medical research and, while the magnitude of the problem remains to be established, it is suspected that many cases of research misconduct pass undetected.

The potential for fraud will always be present. As Broad and Wade remarked: *"Science... is not an idealised interrogation of nature by dedicated servants of truth, but a human process governed by the ordinary human passions of ambition, pride, and greed, as well as by all the well-hymned virtues attributed to men of science."* [44] When presented with the results of mega-trials, the possibility of research misconduct must always be considered. It is a major weakness of large-scale randomised trials that they offer little defence against fraud.

A Waste of Health Care Resources

In an environment of perpetual financial pressures on health care budgets, it is remarkable that the results of mega-trials are accepted, and acted upon, so readily. Guidelines on the management of patients with the common chronic diseases that are based on the results of these studies inevitably lead to a huge waste of scarce resources.

In the case of lipid-lowering drugs, for example, only a very small percentage of patients receiving this treatment will obtain any benefit. For every one million pounds spent on statins, more than

£950,000 will be wasted on patients who – according to the data from mega-trials – would either remain free from problems regardless of treatment or who would develop the outcome despite treatment. Similar estimates apply in the case of ACE inhibitors for ischaemic heart disease and many other drugs used for the long-term management of chronic illnesses.

The case in favour of using these drugs is often supported by economic analyses which purport to show that the financial costs are acceptable. Once again, of course, such claims must be scrutinised. They depend, amongst other things, on the external validity of the mega-trials which has been repeatedly brought into question. Moreover, the motivation of those involved in promoting such treatments must be subjected to examination. For example, the use of these drugs in as broad a population of patients as possible is clearly in the interest of the pharmaceutical companies while, in contrast, restricting treatment to narrow subgroups of patients who would be more likely to benefit would greatly reduce their profits.

The market for prescription drugs is enormous. Worldwide, it exceeded $300 billion in 2000.[48] In the United Kingdom, more than £7 billion is spent on drugs,[20] accounting for more than 15% of total health care expenditure and this proportion has been increasing in recent years. As long as the results of mega-trials continue to tempt the unwary into the widespread use of treatments with at most marginal benefits, the spending on drugs will pursue an inexorably upward trend and resources that might otherwise have been used to produce genuine benefits for patients will continue to be squandered.

Ethical Issues

Nowadays, doctors are encouraged, if not obliged, to provide patients with all the relevant information with which to make informed decisions about their own management.[49] In this climate, it seems appropriate to consider how much detail should be disclosed regarding treatments based on the results of mega-trials.

As discussed earlier, drugs such as statins or angiotensin converting enzyme inhibitors produce very small treatment benefits - indeed, many thousands of patients have to be followed up for years in order to demonstrate differences of a few percent between the drug and placebo. Should patients be informed of this? Should they be told that their chance of any benefit from prolonged treatment is very small? Should they be told that more than 95% of patients who take these drugs derive no benefit whatsoever? Surely, if patients are to participate actively in decisions about their management, then it is crucial that they are aware of these facts.

Whilst it goes without saying that a full description of mega-trials would be impracticable, some indication about the reliability of their data would seem to be essential for any balanced judgment concerning the efficacy of treatment. Should patients, then, be informed about the potential flaws, the widespread low standard of reporting of clinical trials and the questionable external validity – if not in detail, at least in outline? More importantly, should patients be told about the influence of vested interests and its effect on the interpretation and presentation of the data? And should they be made aware of the possibility of both misrepresentation of the data and fraud? Alternatively, of course, doctors could simply impart to their patients a degree of uncertainty with respect to their recommendations, perhaps couched in terms of the imperfections of clinical trials. Given the character of the data from mega-trials, this would at least avoid the temptation to make unfounded claims for knowledge in these matters.

Mega-trials also raise ethical issues in respect of medical practice. Whilst the justification for the widespread use of drugs associated with small treatment differences is often based on the supposed benefits that may be observed in large populations, this argument cannot by itself be used to support treatment in an individual patient. A very large trial showing a statistically significant absolute difference in mortality of 0.3% might support the claim that the widespread use of the drug in a common disease would save thousands of lives but it would hardly justify recommending long-term treatment to an individual patient. Any decision to prescribe treatment must be based solely on the belief that it will be of benefit to the individual concerned.

Interestingly, a recent study from Darlington[50] has shed light on many of these issues. Three-hundred-and-seven individuals participated: two-thirds had a recent admission to coronary care or were receiving long-term, preventive cardiovascular drugs; the remainder had no history of heart disease and were not receiving cardiovascular medication. All subjects completed a questionnaire concerning a hypothetical new drug that reduced the risk of myocardial infarction over a period of five years. One week later, they were interviewed by telephone to determine how large the benefits would have to be for each subject to take long-term medication. The median values of the lowest absolute risk reduction for acceptance of treatment was 20-30%, depending of the patient's history of heart disease. Moreover, three-quarters of the subjects would not take the drug if the benefit were less than 5% over five years. Almost 80% stated that they wanted to be informed of the chance of benefit while only 3.8% knew, even approximately, the benefit to be expected from their current cardiovascular medication; most, in fact, greatly overestimated the benefit.

This study[50] is important because it provides evidence in support of the view that patients are not convinced by the small treatment differences reported by mega-trials. Instead they demand more substantial benefits if they are to be persuaded to take long-term therapy. Moreover, it makes clear that patients want accurate information relating to the benefits of long-term medication. But it also confirms that, at present, few patients are provided with the relevant information. These findings have significant implications particularly in respect of the current recommendations issued by government institutions concerning the management of patients with chronic illnesses such as ischaemic heart disease. As the authors point out: *"... our enthusiasm to lower disease prevalence in the community needs to be tempered by respect for the individual's expectation of drug benefit and a realisation that many are reluctant to take drugs long-term from which they have little chance of benefit."* [50]

Given the importance in contemporary medical practice attributed both to the autonomy of patients and to ensuring that informed consent has been obtained, it is likely that these ethical issues will be a major driving force for change in respect of large-scale randomised trials. If patients were fully informed about all aspects of these studies, then most would be unwilling to accept the recommended treatment. By itself, this would be a salutary lesson for all proponents of mega-trials while the ensuing steep decline in the market for these drugs would prompt a complete re-appraisal of clinical research.

Conclusions

Leaving aside the flawed methodology, large-scale randomised trials have many deleterious consequences. The data are readily open to manipulation, ranging from exaggerated claims to patently misleading conclusions. Such manipulation is facilitated by the excessive latitude for interpretation resulting from marginal treatment differences and disguised by the complexity of the data. These features allow those with a vested interest in the outcome of mega-trials to present the data in the most favourable light. Regulatory authorities and medical institutions are not averse to interpret data selectively while there is little to prevent the pharmaceutical industry from distorting the results in order to maximize their profits.

The vagueness and uncertainty characteristic of the data from mega-trials are the source of the many disputes that nowadays feature in medical journals. It is hardly surprising that medical research is brought into disrepute; if the "gold standard" is unable to deliver clear and unequivocal answers, then how can we have confidence in the results of any medical research?

But mega-trials have further consequences. The failure to provide any substantial defence against fraud – in particular, the absence of any independent mechanism for checking the validity of the results – is a major weakness of the methodology and is of particular concern when the stakes are so high in terms of profit and loss for pharmaceutical companies. The small treatment differences produced by these studies entail that the overwhelming majority of patients receive treatment unnecessarily, resulting in an enormous waste of health care resources. Finally, the special circumstances of mega-trials raise important ethical issues, in terms of both the information given to patients and the decisions made by doctors about treatment based on these studies.

References

1. ASSET study group. Trial of tissue plasminogen activator for mortality reduction in acute myocardial infarction. Anglo-Scandinavian Study of Early Thrombolysis (ASSET). *Lancet* 1988;ii;525-30.

2. ISIS-2 (Second International Study of Infarct Survival) Collaborative Group. Randomised trial of intravenous streptokinase, oral aspirin, both or neither among 17187 cases of suspected acute myocardial infarction: ISIS-2. *Lancet* 1988;2;349-60.

3. The GUSTO Investigators. An international randomised trial comparing four thrombolytic strategies for acute myocardial infarction. *New Eng J Med* 1993;329;673-82.

4. Gruppo Italiano per lo Studio della Sopravvivenza nell'Infarcto Miocardico. GISSI-3: effects of lisinopril and transdermal glyceryl trinitrate singly and together on 6-week mortality and ventricular function after acute myocardial infarction. *Lancet* 1994;343;1115-22.

5. The Heart Outcomes Prevention Evaluation Study Investigators. Effects of an angiotensin-converting-enzyme inhibitor, ramipril, on cardiovascular events in high-risk patients. *New Eng J Med* 2000;342;145-153.

6. Skolbekken JA. Communicating the risk reduction achieved by cholesterol reducing drugs. *Br Med J* 1998;316;1956-8.

7. Altman DG, Schultz KF, Moher D, et al. The revised CONSORT statement for reporting randomised trial: explanation and elaboration. *Ann Intern Med* 2001;134;663-94.

8. Nuovo J, Melnikow J, Chang D. Reporting number needed to treat and absolute risk reduction in randomised controlled trials. *JAMA* 2002;287;2813-4.

9. Slaytor ER & Ward JE. How risks of breast cancer and benefits of screening are communicated to women: analysis of 58 pamphlets. *Br Med J* 1998;317;263-4.

10. Bucher HC, Weinbacher M, Gyr K. Influence of method of reporting study results on decision of physicians to prescribe drugs to lower cholesterol concentration. *Br Med J* 1994;309;761-4.

11. Fahey T, Griffiths S, Peters TJ. Evidence based purchasing: understanding results of clinical trials and systematic reviews. *Br Med J* 1995;311;1056-9.

12. Naylor CD, Chen E, Strauss B. Measured enthusiasm: does the method of reporting trial results alter perceptions of therapeutic effectiveness? *Ann Intern Med* 1992;117;916-21.

13. Elting LS, Martin CG, Cantor SB, et al. Influence of data display formats on physician investigators' decisions to stop clinical trials: prospective trial with repeated measures. *Br Med J* 1999;318;1527-31.]

14. The Long-Term Intervention with Pravastatin in Ischaemic Disease (LIPID) Study Group. Prevention of cardiovascular events and death with pravastatin in patients with coronary heart disease and a broad range of initial cholesterol levels. *New Eng J Med* 1998;339;1349-57.

15. Plehn JF, Davis BR, Sack FM, et al. Reduction of stroke incidence after myocardial infarction with pravastatin. The Cholesterol and Recurrent Events (CARE) Study. *Circulation* 1999;99;216-23.

16. Freemantle N & Hill S. Medicalisation, limits to medicine, or never enough money to go around? *Br Med J* 2002;324;864-5.

17. National Institute for Clinical Excellence. Guidance to the NHS on zanamivir (Relenza). October 1999.

18. Zanamivir for influenza. *Drug and Therapeutics Bulletin* 1999;37(11);81-4.

19. National Institute for Clinical Excellence. Guidance on the use of zanamivir (Relenza) in the treatment of influenza. *NICE Technology Appraisal Guidance* - No. 15. November 2000.

20. Abraham J. The pharmaceutical industry as a political player. *Lancet* 2002;360;1498-502.

21. Collier J, Iheanacho I. The pharmaceutical industry as an informant. *Lancet* 2002;360;1405-9.

22. Kjaergard LL & Als-Nielsen B. Association between competing interests and author's conclusions: epidemiological study of randomised clinical trials published in the BMJ. *Br Med J* 2002;325;249-52.

23. Bodenheimer T. Uneasy alliance – clinical investigators and the pharmaceutical industry. *New Eng J Med* 2000;342;1539-44.

24. Angell M. Is academic medicine for sale? *New Eng J Med* 2000;342;516-8.

25. Friedberg M, Saffran B, Stinson TJ, et al. Evaluation of conflict of interest in economic analyses of new drugs used in oncology. *JAMA* 1999;282;1453-7.

26. Moynihan R. Alosetron: a case study in regulatory capture, or a victory for patients' rights? *Br Med J* 2002;325;592-5.

27. Lievre M. Alosetron for irritable bowel syndrome. *Br Med J* 2002;325;555-6.

28. American Heart Association in collaboration with the International Liaison Committee on Resuscitation and Emergency Medicine. Guidelines 2000 for cardiopulmonary resuscitation and emergency cardiovascular care. Part 7: The era of reperfusion: Section 2: acute stroke. *Circulation* 2000;102 (8 Suppl 1);1204-16.

29. Lenzer J. Alteplase for stroke: money and optimistic claims buttress the "brain attack" campaign. *Br Med J* 2002;324;723-6.

30. Saver JL, Kidwell CS, Starkman S. Commentary: Thrombolysis in stroke: it works! *Br Med J* 2002;324;727-9.

31. Mann H. Uncertainty remains about efficacy. *Br Med J* 2002;324;1581.

32. Solomon RC. Financial information is needed to ensure objectivity. *Br Med J* 2002;324;1582.

33. Hoffman JR. Why were these authors of the commentaries chosen? *Br Med J* 2002;324;1582.

34. Marler JR, Tilley BC, Lu M, et al. Early stroke treatment associated with better outcome: the NINDS rt-PA stroke study. *Neurology* 2000;55;1649-55.

35. Kelch RP. Maintaining the public trust in clinical research. *New Eng J Med* 2002;346;285-7.

36. Editorial. A health scare in the mass media. *Lancet* 2002;359;1079.

37. Antithrombotic Trialists' Collaboration. Collaborative meta-analysis of randomised trials of antiplatelet therapy for prevention of death, myocardial infarction, and stroke in high risk patients. *Br Med J* 2002;324;71-86.

38. Reilly M, Fitzgerald GA. Gathering intelligence on antiplatelet drugs: the view of 30,000 feet. *Br Med J* 2002;324;59-60.

39. Cleland JGF. For debate: Preventing atherosclerotic events with aspirin. *Br Med J* 2002;324;103-5.

40. Gelmon KA, & Olivotto I. The mammography screening debate: time to move on. *Lancet* 2002;359;904-5.

41. Gotzsce PC, Olsen O. Is screening for breast cancer with mammography justifiable? *Lancet* 2000;355;129-34.

42. Horton R. Screening mammography – an overview revisited. *Lancet* 2001;358;1284-5.

43. Horton R. Editor's reply. *Lancet* 2002;359;441-2.

44. Broad W & Wade N. *Betrayers of the Truth*. Oxford University Press. Oxford, 1985.

45. Farthing M, Horton R, Smith R. Research misconduct: Britain's failure to act. *Br Med J* 2000;321;1485-6.

46. Royal College of Physicians of London. Fraud and misconduct in medical research. London: *Royal College of Physicians*, 1991.

47. Misconduct in biomedical research: final consensus statement. In: Nimmo WS (Ed). Joint consensus conference on misconduct in biomedical research. *Proc Roy Coll Physicians Edinb* 2000;30(suppl 7).

48. Henry D & Lexchin J. The pharmaceutical industry as medicines provider. *Lancet* 2002;360;1590-5.

49. Gillon R. Medical ethics: four principles plus attention to scope. *Br Med J* 1994;309;184-8.

50. Trewby PN, Reddy AV, Trewby CS, et al. Are preventive drugs preventive enough? A study of patients' expectation of benefit from preventive drugs. *Clin Med: J Roy Coll Physicians, London* 2002;2;527-33.

VI

TURNING A BLIND EYE IN DEFENCE OF VESTED INTERESTS

In the face of the litany of criticisms levelled against large-scale randomised trials, the widespread, unquestioning acceptance of these studies appears perverse. Why is there so little resistance to such dubious methodology? Why is any challenge so easily snuffed out? Why are the obvious limitations of mega-trials so readily ignored? After all, it is not as if their results have such striking benefits. No doubt, many researchers are driven by a desire to relieve suffering and improve the health of large numbers of people but even those guided by the best of intentions should surely question a methodology that promises so much yet delivers so little. Medical researchers, however, are not alone in failing to address the highly suspect methodology of mega-trials. The entire medical establishment embraces the randomised controlled trial. So, too, do the decision-makers in health care – for example, the Royal Colleges, the NHS management and drug regulatory authorities – as well as the pharmaceutical industry.

The explanation for this collective turning of a blind eye lies in the vested interests that so many diverse groups and institutions have in large-scale randomised trials.

The Medical Establishment

During their clinical training, medical students are introduced to randomised trials. They learn to respect such studies and to trust their results. They become aware of the high esteem in which large-scale randomised trials are held and conversant with the acronyms used to refer to the latest international, multi-centre studies that slip so easily from the tongues of their teachers. By the time they qualify, this methodology is ingrained in their thinking. Thereafter, their beliefs receive nothing but reinforcement. Opening any journal, they are constantly exposed to the hackneyed tribute that randomised trials are the "gold standard" of medical research, articles extolling the virtues of these studies and dismissive arguments against other non-randomised trials. By the time they become involved in medical research, they are steeped in the establishment view of the primacy of randomised trials.

A recent editorial in *The Times*[1] described randomised trials as *"the greatest shibboleth of modern doctoring"*. Indeed, tacit acceptance of the methodology is the *sine qua non* for membership of the medical research community. The randomised controlled trial is a paradigm, a basic feature of medical research, and, as such, is not itself subjected to scrutiny. Those learning to carry out medical research do not study the randomised controlled trial in abstract; instead, they become acquainted with it as if it were a tool and learn to use it in particular situations. But, as for the methodology itself, that is something that is not brought into question. This failure to appraise critically the basic elements of any scientific endeavour is not, though, confined to medical research. As Thomas Kuhn observed, the practice of science will *"...seldom evoke overt disagreement over fundamentals"*.[2] The essential difference, of course, is that science delivers advances with proven practical application whereas mega-trials have no observable benefit.

The uncritical adoption of mega-trials applies not only to those new to medical research but also to the professors and senior lecturers whose careers have depended upon this methodology. In many cases their reputations have been founded on the results of these studies. Many, too, have close links to the pharmaceutical industry which relies on large-scale randomised trials to deliver the ammunition with which to market their products. In some cases, these links involve personal financial gain – investigators may receive thousands of pounds for each patient recruited to a study[3] as well as payments for lectures and expenses for overseas meetings – whilst, in others, they relate to direct funding for their departments. In these circumstances, criticism of large-scale randomised trials is hardly likely to originate from the higher echelons of the medical research community.

The editors of medical journals, too, contribute to the atmosphere of reverence. For example, on the fiftieth anniversary of the first published randomised controlled trial, the *British Medical Journal* devoted an entire issue in celebration of the event.[4] This allegiance continues unabated. Three years later, a leading article in the same journal stated: *"Britain has given the world Shakespeare, Newtonian physics, the theory of evolution, parliamentary democracy – and the randomised controlled trial."* [5] Perhaps it was the festive spirit – it was, after all, the Christmas edition - but, nonetheless, to speak of randomised trials in the same breath as Shakespeare, Newton and Darwin reveals the grossly inflated importance currently bestowed upon this dubious methodology.

Politics, Management and the NHS

Usurping the power of the medical profession

During the final decades of the 20th century, as people lived longer, as the threshold for the diagnosis of diseases decreased, as new and expensive treatments were developed and as the expectations of patients were raised, the pressures on the resources of health care systems increased inexorably and reform became unavoidable. For reform to be possible, however, obstacles had to be removed. And the greatest obstacle was the medical profession. Ever since the inception of the NHS, doctors have been perceived as being too powerful, too independent and too resistant to change.

But, of late, the climate has appeared ideal for a confrontation with the medical profession.

Recent years have not been kind to doctors. Unfortunately, most people are by now familiar with the press photographs of an ashen-faced individual alongside his solicitor on the steps of the General Medical Council - another ignominious exit from the profession as a result of clinical negligence, sexual indiscretions or financial irregularities. And then, of course, there is the television footage of the bearded general practitioner interspersed with images of the cemetery floodlit at the dead of night for the exhumations while all the time estimates of the total number of murdered elderly patients mount. This appalling publicity is grist to the mill for those intent on weakening the medical profession. But it is not enough. A recent survey reported that doctors were regarded as the most trustworthy of all professionals in the United Kingdom.[6] Bad publicity may provide the impetus for appraisal and revalidation but more is needed to take power out of the hands of the medical profession. And what better than to loosen the doctors' claims to be the sole arbiters of the treatment of patients?

Evidence-based medicine

On the surface, evidence-based medicine was introduced in order to improve the quality of health care and to limit expenditure by reducing unnecessary investigations and inappropriate treatment. At another level, though, it allows for a restructuring of the delivery of health care both in terms of limiting clinical freedom of the medical profession and permitting others to perform work normally considered to be the prerogative of doctors.

Evidence-based medicine entails the establishment of an edifice of medical knowledge which may be used to make decisions about the management of patients. For, if recommendations and instructions concerning these decisions are to hold any weight, they must firmly grounded. Inevitably, the evidence base is constructed primarily using the results of randomised controlled trials and their offspring, meta-analyses. Given their universal acceptance, any data derived from them is resistant to challenge. Thus, the randomised trial supplies the foundation for evidence-based medicine. In return, evidence-based medicine reinforces the central role of the randomised trial in providing the most reliable data on which to make clinical decisions. Most articles discussing evidence-based medicine in relation to specific clinical situations include a section on the hierarchy of evidence which gives pride of place to the results from randomised controlled trials and, in particular, to mega-trials. This emphasis on large-scale randomised trials is the Achilles heel of evidence-based medicine.

Guidelines

One of the main components of evidence-based medicine is the production of clinical guidelines, in other words, recommendations concerning the management of particular problems encountered in the delivery of health care. The proliferation of guidelines testifies to their current popularity amongst certain groups in the NHS.

Guidelines are promoted as a means of ensuring that the best treatment is provided for patients. But, regardless of whether or not they actually achieve this outcome, they have other important consequences. They enable the views of decision-makers in the NHS to be imposed on doctors, restricting their clinical freedom; and they supply the grounds for replacing medical staff with other health care professionals. In former times, decisions made by doctors were inaccessible to all but those who had been to medical school. Now, not only do the abstracts of meta-analyses provide instant expertise concerning even the most esoteric of diseases and treatments, but also guidelines may be understood and used by anyone taking the trouble to browse through the flow diagrams and algorithms. And, if it is really the case that medicine can be so easily simplified, then surely many of the decisions formerly the domain of doctors could be left to non-medical staff? This, of course, is precisely what has occurred recently. The assessment of patients in general practice, invasive investigations such as the endoscopic examination of the gastro-intestinal tract, and the management of acutely ill patients with suspected myocardial infarction are nowadays carried out by individuals without a medical qualification. But guidelines disregard much of what is essential to the traditional practice of medicine. They create the illusion that the art of history-taking and examination, the interpretation of the results of investigations, the complex thought processes that lead to the diagnosis and the balanced judgements involved in the management of patients are entirely expendable. And, they encourage the belief that years of clinical experience on a background of lengthy study are dispensible.[7] *"Algorithms that reduce patient care into a sequence of binary decisions often do injustice to the complexity of medicine and the parallel and iterative thought processes inherent in clinical judgment."* [8]

In the past few years, guidelines drop into the letter box almost as often as promotion material for latest lipid-lowering drug or non-steroidal anti-inflammatory agent. Professionally packaged and originating from the relevant learned society, they are sanctioned by the National Institute for Clinical Excellence or one of the Royal Colleges and have a list of contributors bristling with the foremost experts of the day. At a stroke, the contents are welcomed - how could anyone object to the judgment of such august institutions? It is reassuring, however, to know that there are voices of dissent: *"Naive consumers of guidelines accept official recommendations on face value, especially when they carry the imprimatur of prominent professional groups or government bodies."* [8]

Despite their appeal to many sections of the health service, guidelines have numerous drawbacks.[7,8] Their success depends, amongst other things, on the assumptions that the outcomes of trials are reproducible in routine clinical practice and that the widespread adoption of an effective treatment produces optimal treatment for the entire population. Neither of these is supported by clinical experience.[8] In addition, there is little evidence that guidelines actually influence medical practice as reviews suggest that they rarely affect the way in which patients are managed.[9-11] Guidelines are inconvenient and time-consuming, factors which inhibit their use by busy clinicians while the removal of clinical discretion results in resentment and further discourages compliance. Conflicting guidelines produce confusion in clinical practice while flawed guidelines may result in patients receiving the incorrect treatment. In addition, they raise the spectre of possible litigation on the grounds that a doctor failed to comply with the guidelines.[7,8]

These problems, however, fade into the background when attention turns to the validity of the guidelines. Whenever they are based on evidence from large-scale randomised trials, guidelines must be viewed with caution, not just on the grounds of the flaws in the methodology but because of the ease with which the data from mega-trials may be manipulated. It is recognised that the conclusions reached by panels of experts formulating guidelines are subject to bias.[7,8] The case of the recommendations by the American Heart Association for the use of alteplase in patients with acute stroke clearly shows how those with a vested interest may influence the content of guidelines[12] and other studies have reported similar conflicts of interest.[13,14] It seems that most guidelines are produced by experts with financial ties to the pharmaceutical industry. A recent survey of 44 clinical guidelines reported that 87% of authors admitted to such involvement; more than half had been paid to carry out research, more than one-third had been employed by, or were consultants to, pharmaceutical companies and two-thirds had received fees for lecturing.[14] These links were declared in only one of the 44 guidelines. Moreover, even when attention is drawn in the correspondence columns of medical journals to the weaknesses of published studies, little notice is taken of these criticisms when drawing up guidelines.[15] There is little doubt that guidelines may be used by various groups – not only pharmaceutical industry, but government agencies and patient-groups - to promote their interests.

Behind the façade of improving health care, the cult of evidence-based medicine offers a means of reducing costs and curtailing the power of the medical profession. NHS reforms depend, at least in part, on evidence-based medicine which, in turn, depends on the notion of a secure body of knowledge founded on randomised controlled trials. Thus any criticism of the methodology is a direct challenge to health service reforms and, by necessity, must be resisted. To lose the "gold standard" of clinical research would be unthinkable: if the randomised trial were open to question, if guidelines were open to doubt, then there would be no credible argument against the judgement of individual doctors based on years of learning and experience. The illusion of the integrity of the large-scale randomised controlled trial must be protected at all cost.

Allegiance to Randomised Trials

- **University departments**
- **Individual researchers**

- **Politicians**
- **NHS management**

- **Pharmaceutical industry**

The Pharmaceutical Industry

The relationship between randomised controlled clinical trials and the pharmaceutical industry is somewhat paradoxical. On the one hand, clinical trials are viewed as a control mechanism to protect patients from unwarranted claims for efficacy of new drugs. On the other hand, however, large-scale trials are the only means by which the actions of certain drugs may be demonstrated. Thus, clinical trials limit and restrict the pharmaceutical industry while at the same time they alone supply the grounds for the marketing of lucrative drugs used in common diseases. It is clearly in the interest of the pharmaceutical industry for the large-scale randomised controlled trial to remain at the centre of medical research. Indeed, if mega-trials did not exist, then the pharmaceutical industry would have to invent them.

Very few new drugs produce a large therapeutic effect. Many, in fact, are associated with only marginal benefits demonstrated by small absolute differences between the active drug and placebo. Given the requirement on the part of the regulatory authorities for evidence of the efficacy of all new drugs, any challenge to large-scale randomised trials would present a considerable threat to the pharmaceutical industry. For example, without mega-trials, statins – drugs currently prescribed for one in twenty of the American population and responsible for vast profits by the industry – would simply not be marketable because there would be no means of convincing either the regulatory authorities or practicing clinicians of the efficacy of this medication.

Another advantage to the pharmaceutical industry is that once a study is described as a large-scale randomised controlled trial, it receives a stamp of authenticity which tends to inhibit any debate about the results. The mere mention of such studies, whether in promotional material or by the company representative in their sales pitch, is guaranteed to stifle any qualms about claims for the efficacy of their new drug. Furthermore, because of the ease with which the results of mega-trials may be manipulated, the data may be presented in the most favourable light in order to assist the promotion and sales of new drugs.

The absence of any clinically detectable therapeutic effect and the inability of replication to refute the results are of enormous value to the pharmaceutical industry. Apart from minor skirmishes in the correspondence columns of journals with little lasting damage, the results of a published mega-trial are adopted as firm evidence and remain in the literature without serious challenge. Thus, the considerable expense involved in carrying out these studies is well repaid with data that survives for at least as long as the patent for the new drug.

There is, however, a further reason for pharmaceutical companies to favour mega-trials. While alternative approaches to the investigation of new drugs might involve the identification of specific homogeneous groups of patients who would benefit from treatment, this would radically reduce the size of the market for the drug compared with that derived from large-scale randomised trials and, thus, drastically reduce profits. The majority of patients in mega-trials obtain no benefit whatsoever from the medication yet, because the study population is grouped together and no attempt is made to differentiate between those who benefit and those who do not, the results are conveniently applied to the general population with the disease. The pharmaceutical industry has no incentive to identify homogeneous groups of patients in order to focus new treatments on those who would actually benefit; on the contrary, they have every reason to maintain the *status quo* and support mega-trials which greatly expand the market for their wares.

The *raison d'etre* of every pharmaceutical company is to make money for their shareholders. And they are very successful. In 2001, the pharmaceutical industry was the most profitable sector of the US economy with the top ten companies increasing their profits by 32%, from $28 to $37 billion.[16] Moreover, total spending on prescription drugs has increased steeply in recent years, almost doubling between 1997 and 2001 to $155 billion.[17] Drugs used for long-term therapy in chronic diseases afflicting many in western societies account for much of the profits of these companies and, since their efficacy is established predominantly by large-scale randomised trials, the success of the pharmaceutical industry is heavily dependent on this methodology.[18]

It is obvious that the pharmaceutical industry has the motivation for ensuring that their new products perform well in large-scale randomised trials. It also has the means at its disposal. Governments, intent on supporting business, maintain close links with the pharmaceutical industry[19] while feeble regulatory authorities, financially dependent on the industry, offer little opposition to the marketing of new drugs.[19,20] Furthermore, the pharmaceutical industry is heavily involved in medical research, especially in respect of funding; it is often the driving force behind the initiation of clinical trials and responsible for the design of the studies; in many instances, it participates in data collection and analysis; in addition, pharmaceutical companies choose – and have financial links with - the investigators.[19] In the murky world of mega-trials, with equivocal data open to easy manipulation, the pharmaceutical industry is ideally placed to influence the outcome of clinical research. In this context, it is pertinent to recall that studies sponsored by pharmaceutical companies are more likely to deliver favourable results compared with independent research.[19,21,22]

Conclusions

Government, regulatory authorities and health service planners, university professors and researchers, as well as the pharmaceutical industry, have every reason to encourage the current allegiance to the large-scale randomised trial. Whether to provide a foundation for reforms, to preserve reputations and protect personal financial gain, or to secure future profits, maintenance of the *status quo* with respect to mega-trials is mandatory. Too much has been invested in this methodology for questions about its validity to be given even so much as a fleeting acknowledgement. The ease with which such questions may be dismissed, however, speaks volumes for the poverty of much of what passes for medical research. Gone is the search for knowledge; instead, the establishment settles for the froth that emerges from the mega-trials. Sophistry, it seems, is more than simply tolerated; nowadays, it is embraced - provided, of course, that it serves the interests of those in power. It is an old, old story, as Schopenhauer recognised: *"Party interests are vehemently agitating the pens of so many pure lovers of wisdom... Truth is certainly the last thing they have in mind... Governments make of philosophy a means of serving their state interests, and scholars make of it a trade."* [23]

References

1. Editorial. NICE Decisions: Bringing rational judgment to the NHS. *The Times* Tuesday, 13th August 2002.

2. Kuhn T. *The Structure of Scientific Revolutions.* University of Chicago Press; Chicago, 1962.

3. Rao JN & Cassia LJS. Ethics of undisclosed payments to doctors recruiting patients in clinical trials. *Br Med J* 2002;325;36-7.

4. The randomised controlled trial at fifty. *Br Med J* 1998;317;1167-1246.

5. Smith R, Chalmers I. Britain's gift: a "Medline" of synthesised evidence. *Br Med J* 2001;323;1437-8.

6. Kmietovicz Z. R.E.S.P.E.C.T. – why doctors are still getting enough of it. *Br Med J* 2002;324;11.

7. Haycox A, Bagust A, Walley T. Clinical guidelines - the hidden costs. *Br Med J* 1999;318;391-3.

8. Woolf SH, Grol R, Hutchinson A, et al. Potential benefits, limitations, and harms of clinical guidelines. *Br Med J* 1999;318;527-30.

9. Freemantel N, Harvey E, Grimshaw JM, et al. The effectiveness of printed educational materials in changing the behaviour of health care professionals. In: Cochrane Collaboration. *Cochrane Library* Issue 3;1996.

10. Bero L, Grilli R, Grimshaw JM, et al. The Cochrane Effective Practice and Organisation of Care Review group. *Cochrane database of systematic reviews,* 1998.

11. Feder G, Eccles M, Grol R, et al. Using clinical guidelines. *Br Med J* 1999;318;728-30.

12. Lenzer J. Alteplase for stroke: money and optimistic claims buttress the "brain attack" campaign. *Br Med J* 2002;324;723-6.

13. Lexchin J. Don't bite the hand that feeds you. *West J Med* 1999;171;238-9.

14. Choudhry NK, Stelfox HT, Detsky AS. Relationships between authors of clinical practice guidelines and the pharmaceutical industry. *JAMA* 2002;287;612-7.

15. Horton R. Postpublication criticism and shaping of clinical knowledge. *JAMA* 2002;287;2843-7.

16. Gottlieb S. Drug companies maintain "astounding" profits. *Br Med J* 2002;324;1054.

17. Editorial. Just how tainted has medicine become? *Lancet* 2002;359;1167.

18. Henry D & Lexchin J. The pharmaceutical industry as a medicines provider. *Lancet* 2002;360;1590-5.

19. Collier J & Iheanacho I. The pharmaceutical industry as an informant. *Lancet* 2002;360;1405-9.

20. Abraham J. The pharmaceutical industry as a political player. *Lancet* 2002;360;1498-502.

21. Davidson R. Source of funding and outcome of clinical trials. *J Gen Intern Med* 1986;1; 155-8.

22. Kjaergard LL & Als-Nielsen B. Association between competing interests and authors' conclusions: epidemiological study of randomised clinical tials published in the BMJ. *Br J Med* 2002;325;249-52.

23. Schopenhauer A. Quoted in: *The Open Society and its Enemies* by KR Popper. Published by Routledge and Kegan Paul, London, 1966 (Fifth Edition); Vol II, Chap 12, page 33.

VII

BUILDING A HOUSE OF CARDS

When a doctor recommends a drug on the basis of the results of a large-scale randomised trial, does he *know* that the treatment works? Does he, for example, feel as confident about the drug working as he does about statements such as "atropine dilates the pupils" or "noradrenaline increases the blood pressure"? Is he certain that the drug works in the same way that he is certain that dilute hydrochloric acid turns blue litmus red? He would wager his house on the truth of the statement that insulin lowers the blood sugar level but would he be so willing to risk that amount on the results of a mega-trial? The contrast in each instance could not be more obvious: on the one hand, we have the vague, uncertain generalisations from mega-trials; on the other, we have precise, reliable generalisations derived from the scientific method.

To know that a causal generalisation about the natural world is true, we must be able to provide an account of how we know it is true. We must be acquainted with the objects involved in the generalisation and identify them without error. We must be in a position to supply evidence in the form of direct observations of the phenomenon. And we must be able to show how the phenomenon is consistent with, and supported by, other established knowledge and theory. Only if these conditions are satisfied, can we claim knowledge of causal relationships. However, the more we scrutinise mega-trials, the more we see that they fail to comply with these conditions. It seems that mega-trials shun the search for knowledge and settle instead for meddling with sophistry.

Knowledge and Common Sense – a Recipe for Success

Consider the case of a patient complaining of progressively worsening pain in the right hip associated with restricted movements; examination suggests disease of the hip joint and an X-ray shows the typical features of advanced osteoarthritis. In these circumstances, the orthopaedic surgeon's statement to the patient that she will benefit from total hip replacement is fully justified. It is, for example, is founded on anatomy and pathology: his knowledge of these subjects allows him to interpret the clinical features and radiological appearances – in other words, to localise the problem accurately and to be confident that it accounts for the symptoms and signs. The natural history of the disease is well established; there are, for instance, no cases of spontaneous resolution and he may, therefore, be certain of the poor outcome without surgical intervention. The development of a prosthetic joint is dependent both upon a detailed knowledge of the anatomy of the hip as well as physics and chemistry, all of which are reliable in these matters. And, of course, his conviction that surgery will be successful is based on the extensive literature relating to similar operations over many years, together with his own personal experience in this field. Finally, there is a transparent, readily understood link between the problem causing the patient's symptoms – namely, the diseased joint – and the treatment by joint replacement. While the skills of the surgeon and the technical expertise involved in the development of the prosthesis are to be admired, the theory on which the treatment is based is no more complicated than that of carpentry.

General surgery, too, uses basic principles to great effect. A patient who presents with a short history of severe colicky abdominal pain, profuse vomiting, marked gaseous distension with increased bowel sounds, and dilated loops of small bowel on X-rays, has intestinal obstruction which, if accompanied by a tender, inflamed mass in the groin, is due to a strangulated hernia. In this situation, the surgeon would be justified in informing the patient that an operation is in their best interest. His knowledge of anatomy and gastro-intestinal physiology explains the complex of symptoms and signs, as well as the radiological appearances. The natural history of a strangulated hernia indicates that the mortality without surgery would be high. His own experience, in addition to that of countless other surgeons, testifies to the beneficial outcome from surgery. Moreover, as in the case of the total hip replacement, there is the straightforward link between the problem – obstruction of the small bowel – and its treatment. The theory underlying the treatment is no more difficult to understand than plumbing: problems resulting from blocked tubes may be resolved by removing the obstruction. So much of surgery involves this simple principle – from infantile pyloric stenosis to biliary tract obstruction due to gallstones, and from renal failure due to benign prostatic hypertrophy to an embolus occluding the femoral artery.

A patient with slowly progressive blindness is examined and found to have large, bilateral cataracts. The decision by the ophthalmic surgeon to recommend operation is well founded. Being directly visible, the lesions are easily localised. The physics of light, together with the anatomy and physiology of the eye, allow an understanding of the way in which the pathology produces its clinical manifestations. The lesions do not resolve without treatment and the outcome of surgical intervention is well established. Once again, however, it is the obvious link between the problem and the treatment that is the foundation for success.

There are many other examples of surgical treatment based on simple theory. A subdural haematoma or a meningioma compress the adjacent brain tissue and impair function, just as a prolapsed intervertebral disc damages the spinal cord; blood, tumour or disc may be removed with beneficial effects. A large pneumothorax or pleural effusion result in collapse of the adjacent lung while a pericardial effusion compromises ventricular function; in each case, aspiration leads to rapid improvement. Once again, the principle behind the disorder is clear - pressure on tissues produces damage which may be reversed if the abnormality is promptly removed.

Factors involved in successful treatment

- **Identification and localisation of the disease**
- **Close relationship between the lesion and symptoms**
- **Knowledge of the natural history of the disease**
- **Knowledge of the previous efficacy of treatment**
- **Obvious link between the disease and the treatment**

All of these examples have features in common which, taken together, explain why we are entitled to feel confident about the diagnosis and the benefit of treatment. The lesion is capable of being defined precisely and is clearly localised. Moreover, the nature and site of the lesion account for the patient's symptoms – they are consistent with a disturbance in the anatomy and physiology of that region. The natural history of the disease is firmly established and is such that spontaneous resolution would not occur; hence, there is a stable background against which to judge the efficacy of treatment. The treatments have been used in innumerable patients over long periods of time with high rates of success. Furthermore, there is a straightforward and transparent link between the clinical problem and the treatment. Thus, if a randomised trial were to be performed in these clinical situations, it would be likely to show a huge absolute treatment difference, with no improvement in untreated patients compared to a successful outcome in the overwhelming majority of those undergoing surgery. However, randomised trials, even if ethically permissible, are not needed. We *know* that the treatment works. We have an acceptable degree of homogeneity in respect of the outcome for both untreated and treated patients; the requirements for resemblance and regularity are present. In addition, the background knowledge and theory are sound, in terms of both the relationship between the lesion and the clinical manifestations and that between the lesion and its treatment. Finally, since all of these examples include patients with active clinical symptoms, the effect of treatment may be demonstrated in the individual cases.

Ultimately, the success of these surgical treatments is founded on the scientific method. And it is the scientific method that justifies the claims that we know that the treatment works. There is, though, another aspect of these examples from the field of surgery that should not be overlooked. The arguments on which these treatments are based are entirely in line with common sense. In other words, the reasoning involved is consistent with the approach to causal relationships in our daily lives. This, of course, should come as no surprise. *"Science is nothing but trained and organised common sense, differing from the latter only as a veteran may differ from a raw recruit: and its methods differ from those of common sense only in so far as the guardsman's cut and thrust differ from the manner in which a savage wields his club."* [1] There is surely a strong element of truth in Huxley's words. After all, there is a shared logic between the scientific method and common sense, both arguing according to the principles of induction and both using the same method of causal inference. Common sense, though, is the last thing that sits comfortably in the presence of large-scale randomised trials.

Without Knowledge or Common Sense – a Recipe for Failure

Faced with the murky data from large-scale randomised trials, the physician could be forgiven for casting an envious eye in the direction of his surgical colleagues. If only he could muster arguments of the calibre of those in favour of total hip replacement, surgery for intestinal obstruction or removal of cataracts; if only he could project such clarity of purpose; if only he could invoke common sense; and, if only he could display knowledge. But cogent arguments, clarity and common sense – these are not attributes which stem from mega-trials. And neither, for that matter, is knowledge.

How much do we really know about the subject matter of any large-scale randomised trial? The decision to perform this type of study is by itself testament to the very limited state of knowledge. It implies, for example, that there is insufficient information available to enable the identification of a group of patients who are homogeneous with respect to the outcome without treatment - indeed, unless this were the case, there would be no requirement for randomisation. And, it indicates that the treatment is expected to prevent the outcome in only a proportion of patients, in other words, that the link between the disease and the proposed treatment is tenuous. Thus, even before the first patient is recruited and before one iota of data is collected, we may be sure that the eventual results will be clouded by uncertainty.

How do we know that the mega-trial has achieved internal validity? For instance, at every point in the randomisation process, errors may occur that disrupt the equal distribution of relevant variables. Such is the complexity of mega-trials, it is not always possible to be certain that the random distribution has been either initially achieved or maintained throughout the study. Even a minor disruption of the randomisation process may account for the small treatment difference. But, given that mega-trials are multi-centre – and often multi-national – involving many thousands of patients, how can any one individual be certain that all of the conditions for internal validity have been satisfied?

Do we know that the treatment based on the results of a mega-trial will be of benefit to an individual patient? All large-scale randomised trials may justifiably be said to yield one item of knowledge: since all such studies entail a small treatment difference, it follows necessarily that they all support the statement the vast majority of patients receives no benefit from the treatment. Given this, we cannot without contradiction claim that we know that the treatment will benefit any individual patient.

Do we know that the use of treatment based on mega-trials will benefit the wider population of patients? In view of the application of selection criteria, it is undeniable that there are differences between patients recruited to these studies and those who are excluded, while the relevance of these differences to the outcome of trials is well documented. Furthermore the conditions of any trial are different from those in routine clinical practice. There are, therefore, sound reasons for asserting that we cannot know that the treatment will be of benefit to the wider population of patients.

Do we know that the data from mega-trials has not been manipulated? And do we know that the study does not involve fraud? Data manipulation is commonplace in the medical literature while research misconduct is of particular concern in the context of large-scale randomised trials. Those with a vested interest have the motive, the opportunity and the means to ensure that results favourable to their cause will be delivered by mega-trials. Furthermore, the failure of the normal checks and balances in science provided by replication, together with the absence of any clinical observations that might bring the results of a trial into question, suggest that fraud is likely to pass unnoticed. The conditions surrounding mega-trials are fertile ground for fraud. In the circumstances, we cannot be sure that the data are not the product of research misconduct.

How do we know that the methodology of mega-trials is valid? Science is characterised by sound background theory and knowledge, homogeneous references classes and regularity in respect of the phenomenon under investigation, which, together, account for its striking success. Mega-trials, in contrast, lack all of these features and this explains their failure to deliver any worthwhile results. The differences between the two methodologies – in particular, the different approaches to causal inference - are so great as to militate against the claim that mega-trials are founded on the scientific method. If, however, this is the case, then mega-trials require an alternative justification - in other words, they have to show that their results are valid. But, while science can demonstrate the validity of its methodology by reference to direct observations of the practical applications of its theories, no such options are open to mega-trials. Without an independent process of verification, we must conclude that the methodology is without any firm foundation. We simply do not know whether the methodology of mega-trials is valid.

The "No Alternative" Argument

Critics of the current approach to medical research are frequently challenged on the grounds that there is no alternative to the large-scale randomised trial. This argument, however, fails on a number of accounts.

Given that the criticism of mega-trials is that the methodology is flawed, it is irrelevant to this argument to reply with the assertion that there is no alternative. Defenders of mega-trials must address the issues directly and demonstrate that the criticisms are invalid rather than indulge in specious arguments.

Even if it were the case that there was no alternative to mega-trials, this would not support the conclusion that a flawed methodology should be used to investigate the efficacy of drug treatments. Surely, in these circumstances, it would be better to do nothing than to subject patients to treatment based on an unproven methodology? In this context, it is worth noting the inconvenience of long-term therapy, with the daily reminders to the patient of their illness, not to mention the continual exposure to potential adverse drug reactions. Moreover, abandoning such treatments would avoid the waste of health care resources and allow the savings to be channelled into areas of care with proven efficacy.

There is a strong element of circularity in the "no alternative" argument. It assumes, for instance, that the value of treatments based on mega-trials is established and that patients would be worse off without this methodology. But this, of course, is only true if the methodology is valid – in other words, if we accept the very issue being contested.

It is, though, simply not the case that there is no alternative to mega-trials. The clues to the solution were given by Bacon in the Age of Reason and by Hume in the Enlightenment. Instead of accepting the extreme heterogeneity characteristic of large-scale trials, we should place more emphasis on the identification of relevant variables present in the background phenomenon by studying the subgroups of patients who actually develop the outcome under control conditions, in other words, in untreated patients. Step-by-step, more homogeneous groups of patients would be available for recruitment to clinical trials. Drugs would then be tested, this time repeating the process of stepwise identification of relevant variables in respect of the outcome during treatment. This approach, which is consistent with classical Baconian induction, would tend to produce more homogeneous study populations, thus allowing trials of new drugs to demonstrate large, clinically meaningful treatment differences. It would, however, be contrary to the guidelines and national standards that ensure that the majority of patients receiving statins, for example, do so without any expectation of benefit. And it would not find favour with the pharmaceutical industry which relies on the huge markets created by mega-trials. Defenders of the *status quo* would, no doubt, assert that it is not possible to identify the relevant variables to enable the creation of more homogeneous populations. Yet this is a sad indictment of current medical research and ought to provide the impetus for change.

A House of Cards

The reputation of medicine is grounded in the many advances which occurred throughout the 20th century. These advances – in surgery, anaesthetics and various fields of medicine – were the result of research based on the scientific method. But the edifice of medical knowledge, accumulated with enormous effort over many years, is now tainted by the products of large-scale randomise trials. For all the accolades bestowed upon them, mega-trials are permeated with uncertainty. Wherever we look, we stumble across nothing but a morass of murky data, unsubstantiated claims and dubious inferences. Can we be sure, for instance, that a mega-trial satisfies the criteria for internal validity? No. Are the results likely to be of any tangible benefit to an individual patient? No. Can the claims for treatment of the wider population be sustained? No. Are we certain that there has been no manipulation of data by those with a vested interest in the outcome? No. Can we confidently exclude fraud? No. Can we trust this method of causal inference? No. The questions raised by mega-trials are endless but the answers are usually the same.

Yet, despite the blatant flaws, mega-trials not only survive, but thrive. It is, of course, easy to be beguiled by the logic of randomisation. It is easy to be mesmerised by the Byzantine theories of statisticians. It is also easy to be fooled by the facade of scientific respectability. But, perhaps the easiest deception is to believe that this methodology eradicates the problems encountered in clinical research. As Julius Caesar observed: *Fere libenter homines id quod volunt credunt* (Men are nearly always willing to believe what they wish).[2] A more cynical explanation, however, is that mega-trials flourish because they serve the vested interests of those involved, openly or covertly, in the outcome of medical research.

The time has surely come to admit that this methodology is unsound. This regrettable state of affairs, of course, could so easily have been avoided if those involved in medical research had listened more attentively to Hume:*"... all kinds of reasoning from causes to effects are founded on two particulars, viz. the constant conjunction of any two objects in all past experience, and the resemblance of a present object to any one of them... If you weaken either the union or resemblance, you weaken the principle of transition, and of consequence that belief, which arises from it.*" [3]

Large-scale randomised trials are deeply flawed. They deliver nothing but a weak shadow of therapeutic benefit, a pretence of efficacy to fool the unwary and the means by which those with little interest in either the integrity of medical research or genuine improvements in health care inflate their reputations and maximise their profits. Time is likely to show that what is being built on the flimsy foundations of mega-trials is nothing more than a house of cards.

References

1. Huxley TE. *Collected Essays* (1893-4).

2. Julius Caesar. *De Bello Gallico* I, iii, 18.

3. Hume D. *A Treatise of Human Nature (1739)*. Edited by EC Mossner. Penguin Books Ltd, Middlesex, England, 1987. Bk I; Part III; Sect XII; P192.

INDEX

Index

Index

scepticism 11
Schopenhauer, A. 119
science 18-32, 57-58, 66, 71, 75-78, 128
scientific knowledge 122-126
scientific method 3, 18-31, 74, 77-78
selection criteria 46-47, 51, 67
Shakespeare, W. 111
small treatment effect 3, 57, 59, 66, 69-74, 79, 89, 101, 117, 127
Snow, J. 63
statistics 42
statistical theory of causation 62-66
subjunctive conditionals 65
Susser, M. 63-64

temporal priority
theory 20, 21, 23, 29-32, 57, 76, 87, 127

universal generalisations 27
US Food & Drug Administration 93

variative induction 19, 25-27, 44
vested interests 47-48, 90, 92, 93-96, 109-121, 131

Wade, N. 97-99
waste of health resources 83, 99-100

Printed in the United Kingdom
by Lightning Source UK Ltd.
9590700001B